Copyright © 1994 Times Mirror International Publishers Limited
Published in 1994 by Mosby–Wolfe, an imprint of Times Mirror International Publishers Limited
Printed by Grafos S.A. Arte sobre papel, Barcelona, Spain.
ISBN 0 7234 19914 (Cased); 07234 20262 (Limp)
1st Edition 1984, Copyright © D. W. Beaven, S.E. Brooks 1984
Published by Wolfe Medical Publications Ltd 1984

For full details of all Times Mirror International Publishers Limited titles please write to Times Mirror International Publishers Limited, Lynton House, 7–12 Tavistock Square, London WC1H 9LB, England.

A CIP catalogue record for this book is available from the British Library.

Library of Congress Cataloging-in-Publication Data has been applied for.

Contents

Acknowledgements

We freely acknowledge our great debt of gratitude to colleagues and registrars over the last 25 years, who brought to our notice many of the nails illustrated in this small guide. Our original collection of 1000 nail patients and normals was the inspiration of Sally Collins, Charge Nurse and Manager of the Professional Medical Unit in Christchurch during most of this period.

Earlier, dermatological colleagues Allan Muir and Derek Lardner gave help and advice, and, more recently, we are particularly indebted to Dr Kenneth MacDonald, Head of Dermatology Services, and his three colleagues for making slides readily available.

Richard Winder, Principal of the New Zealand National Podiatry School, and Greg Coyle, a fellow Councillor, generously made available many of the original toenail illustrations.

Dr James Marshall of Templeton Centre rendered invaluable help in collecting examples from his large group of intellectually disabled patients.

Above all, we have been grateful to a series of professional colleagues in the Audio-Visual and Photographic Departments at Christchurch and Princess Margaret Hospitals, particularly Mrs Fiona Van Oyen, medical illustrator at the Princess Margaret Hospital, for her skill and help in completing the drawings, and Messrs Pengelly (Nelson), Louise Goosen and John Main (Wellington), who assisted with slides.

The following individual specialists and academic staff in Christchurch, Wellington, Dunedin and Auckland have lent slides from their own teaching collections for this edition: Drs Bailey, Barnie, Brownlie, Begg, Ellis-Pegler (Auckland), Darlow, Davis, Janus, McLeod, MacDonald, Moller, O'Donnell, Swainson, Ikram and Hay, and Professors Ahija (India), Donald, Colls, Espiner, Pomare, Morton, Sainsbury and North.

Volunteers, medical students and many departmental colleagues up and down this country, too numerous to name, have assisted. In a growing era of shared knowledge and consent, we remain greatly in the debt of those who patiently agreed to have their nails photographed and appear in this book. Without their help and cooperation, this teaching and diagnostic guide would not have been possible.

Preface

The continuing neglect of careful nail examination in a growing era of better and widely used technology is to be regretted. Such a valuable source of 10 nail sites in people of all countries allows the alert and curious observer to observe swiftly many facets of the health personality and general medical disorders in the person being greeted for the first time. As the health worker, doctor or nurse is introduced to the patient or client, his or her observation of the condition of the patient's nails may lead to a further follow-up examination.

In this second edition, the emphasis is once again entirely for the non-specialist dermatologist. Ninety-nine per cent of the pictures in this edition illustrate findings from examination of general patients or that may be observed in normal people seen in general practice, the ambulant care areas or in general hospital beds.

The first English language edition of this small visual aid to assist in discovering the underlying cause of abnormal nails was published in 1985. Between then and 1989, the focus on nail appearances in the world literature has been primarily on changes produced in association with generalised ectodermal or skin diseases. From 1988 to 1993, a careful review of the world literature (where abstracts have been in English) has shown an increasing interest in the value of nail appearances in clinical diagnosis. This has grown from about 70 papers a year on the human nail, where the primary interest is on appearance or diagnosis, to 128 papers on this subject between 1992 and 1993. In the last five years, there has been a predominance of papers indicating a growing interest in coloured nails and dystrophies related to drug usage, also a marked increase of interest in specialised diagnostic aids such as video microscopy, various forms of capillaroscopy and high-resolution MR imaging to aid diagnosis. The last two years have seen the emergence of a new emphasis on antigenic staining and analysis of trace elements in nail clippings, and the beginnings of a new development of molecular biology on nail material using CDNA and genomic cloning techniques.

In order for a referral to a specialist nail physician or dermatologist with the skills to use these new techniques, it is now more important than 10 years ago for the practising family doctor, independent nurse practitioner, podiatrist or specialist in other disciplines to recognise that any nail changes present are a deviation from normal, and not merely a result of ageing.

In adding to a wider range of commonly occurring nail appearances in this second edition, the opportunity to review the world literature over the last 4–5 years has allowed the inclusion of references to more common disorders, or significant trends in the fields of nail diagnosis.

The art and science of good-quality health care depends upon skill and training. We hope that this collection of photographs will assist in identifying those common disorders which will help in swifter diagnosis, better reassurance and the confidence to refer onwards to the appropriate specialist practitioner. Above all, it is our conviction that developing a life-long curiosity about abnormal findings and their possible meaning is enhanced by looking at the fingernails of every client or patient.

Introduction to Second Edition

We are gratified that commonly occurring disorders selected from about 1000 photographs in 1984 are still commonly seen in 1994. The motive for producing a small diagnostic aid for senior students, practitioners, podiatrists and others was the belief that an alert observation of the nails was possible in all countries and in all people. The nails are a unique site of specialised keratin material, and abnormalities demonstrate the physical status of health over the previous few months. Translations of the first edition into four languages confirm this viewpoint.

Valuable comments from reviewers, friends and many correspondents have been incorporated in this rewritten nail guide, which we hope will be more useable.

Chapter 1

The Normal Nail

Fingernails and toenails have evolved over more than 300 million years. As well as protecting the highly sensitive and touch-specialised tips of the fingers and toes, they improve the fine "picking" movements and sensitive function of pairs of digits. They are less used now for some offensive and defensive activities.

In embryonic life, the inward turning of the developing skin forms the specialised nail-producing organs. The nail plate, the largest and most visible sheet of specialised keratin, is a vital indicator of health events over the previous months. At the base of the nail, the matrix cells form the specialised keratin sheet and push it forward to the free margin, recording for those who are curious enough to examine the nails a unique story of past and present health events.

The forward growth of the nail plate, dependent on end arteries supplying the matrix cells and influenced by end pulp shunts, finishes at the yellow line (Figure 1). The nail plate beyond the yellow line leads to the free edge, which is of variable length and thickness, depending upon frequency of cutting and occupation. The area under the free edge is called the hyponychium.

The nail bed consists of a deeper portion or dermis and the outer section or epidermis (Figure 2). The section of the nail bed under the proximal nail fold, the cuticle and the lunula is also often referred to as the matrix. The dermis of the nail bed is arranged in longitudinal grooves and ridges. The epidermis is thickened and gradually passes into the nail with swelling of matrix cells, nucleolysis and subsequent shrinkage. The lunula or white "half moon" at the base or proximal end of the nail is particularly smooth, flat and shiny.

The whiteness of the lunula or

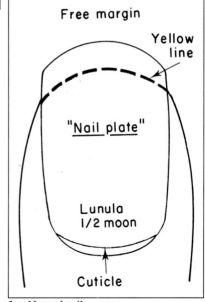

1 Normal nail.

Free margin

Yellow line

"Nail plate"

Lunula 1/2 moon

Cuticle

"half moon" and its aetiology still remains somewhat controversial. Certainly the degree to which the cuticle or proximal end of the nail is regularly pushed back, or "manicured", determines the visibility and size of the lunula (Figure **3**).

In certain chromosomal abnormalities the lunula is absent, i.e., Monosomia 4, and it is seen to be diminished in Trisomy 21. As better DNA

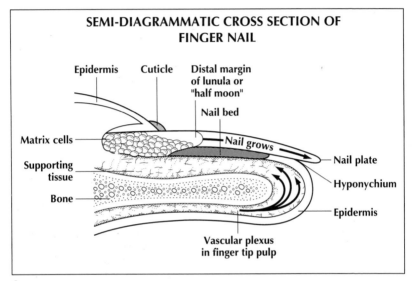

2

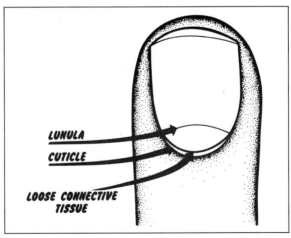

3

probes are developed, we are likely to see identifiers around the nail apparatus as visual markers of underlying genetic abnormalities (*see Chapter 12*).

At the edges of the nail, the skin turns into the nail folds. This junctional area between skin and nail is known as the nail groove. The outer end of the nail groove is important in the great toe because of the frequency of "ingrowing". At the proximal end of the nail is the eponychium, with its loose free border or cuticle.

A few studies of the composition of the nails show high concentrations of sulphur and selenium and moderately high levels of calcium and potassium, but trace element losses from nails are small. The association between trace elements from fingernail clippings to common disorders, occupation and smoking has recently been noted (Sukamar and Subramanian, 1992).

References

1. Cohen, P. R. Geriatric nail disorders: diagnosis and treatment. *Journal of the American Academy of Dermatology,* 1992, **26** (4), 521–31.
2. Ditre, C. M. & Howe, N. R. Surgical anatomy of the nail unit. *Journal of Dermatological Surgery & Oncology,* 1992, **18** (8), 665–71.
3. Dykyj, J. D. Anatomy of the nail. *Clin. Podiatr. Med. Surgery,* 1989, **6** (2), 215–28.
4. Forslind, B. On the structure of the normal nail. A scanning electron microscope study. *Archives fur Dermatologishe Forschung,* 1975, **251**, 199.
5. Harrison, W. W. & Clemena, G. G. Survey analysis of trace elements in human fingernails by spark source mass spectrometry. *Clinica Chimica Acta,* 1972, **36**, 485.
6. Lewin, K. The normal finger nail. *British Journal of Dermatology*, 1961, **77**, 421.
7. Runne, U. The human nail: structure, growth and pathological changes. *Current Problems in Dermatology,* 1981, **9**, 102.
8. Sukumar, A. & Subramanian, R. Elements in hair and nails of residents from a village adjacent to New Delhi. Influence of place of occupation and smoking habits. *Biological Trace Element Research,* 1992, **34** (1), 99–105.
9. Sukumar, A. & Subramanian, R. Elements in hair and nails of urban residents of New Delhi CHD, hypertensive, and diabetic cases. *Biological Trace Elements Research,* 1992, **34** (1), 89–97.
10. Vellar, O. D. Composition of human nail substance. *American Journal of Clinical Nutrition,* 1970, **23**, 1272.
11. Zook, E. G., Van Beek, A. L., Russell, R. C. & Beatty, M. E. Anatomy and physiology of the perionychium: a review of the literature and anatomic study. *Journal of Hand Surgery,* 1980, **5** (6), 528.

Blood Supply

The two digital arteries run on the sides of the fingers as do the returning dorsal arteries from the finger pulp. This means that earliest changes in the blood supply or nutrients to the nails will be seen first in the centre of the nail at the base, or proximal, part of the nail.

The central portion of the nail bed may also be involved, as nail thickness is added from the ventral surface well down the nail. Thus, central lesions from blood supply or nutrient deficiency will become exaggerated towards the free edge of the nail.

As these two end terminal digital arteries run on the palmar (ventral) or touch side of the finger, they give off small branches to form a rich cruciate network or anastomosis at the terminal finger pulp (Figures **4** and **5**).

Here are the very important arterior-venous capillary shunts partially under nervous control and partially controlled by increasingly recognised circulating kinins. The physiology of these digital capillary shunts allows blood to proceed through the fingertip pulp and return to the nail matrix area by two dorsal arteries; this has been well demonstrated by Flint (1955). These capillary shunts terminate in a further dorsal anastomosis, which also receives blood from the branches of the digital arteries mentioned before. Thus, the base of the nail bed and matrix cells can, when the terminal capillary pulps are open, receive a double blood supply with relative increased activity of the cells. This accounts for the overgrowth or sponginess seen in clubbing of the fingernails. Because of these collateral vessels near the fingertip, the finger pulp and the nail beds seldom show much ischaemia.

Recent papers have emphasised the accessibility and value of microscopic studies on the nail fold capillaries in a variety of disorders.

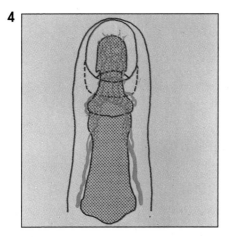

4 Dorsal view of blood supply.

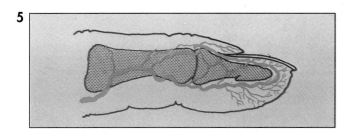

5 Lateral view of blood supply (adapted from Flint). Note supply of matrix via capillary fingertip shunt.

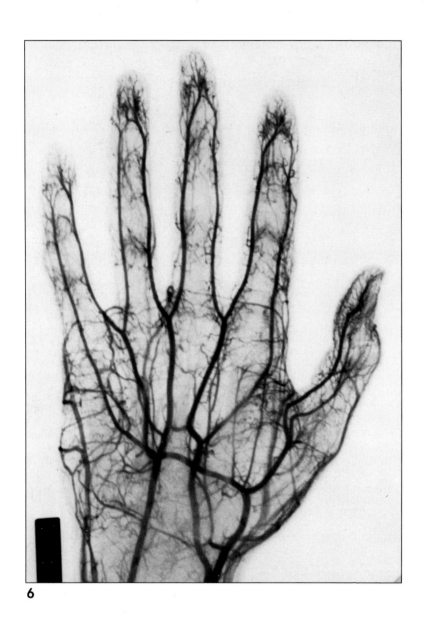

6

6 Angiogram of normal hands showing arterial plexus at fingertips.

7 Close-up of fingertip and nail bed plexus (normal). These are from a normal hand and normal angiogram.

7

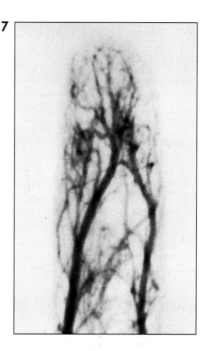

References

1. Clementz, B. A., Iacono, W. G., Ficken, J. & Beiser, M. A family of study of nailfold plexus visibility in psychotic disorders. *Biological Psychiatry*, 1992, **31** (4), 378–90.
2. Flint, M. H. Some observations on the vascular supply of the nail bed and terminal segments of the finger. *British Journal of Plastic Surgery*, 1955, **8**, 186.
3. Gasser, P. & Berger W. Nailfold video microscopy and local cold test in type I diabetes. *Angiology*, 1992, **43** (5), 395–400.
4. Joyal, F., Choquette, D., Roussin, A., Levington, C. & Senecal, J. L., Evaluation of the severity of systemic sclerosis by nailfold capillary microscopy in 112 patients. *Angiology*, 1992, **43** (3, Pt 1), 203–10.
5. Norton, L.A. Incorporation of the thymidine–methyl H^3 and glycine 2 H^3 in the nail matrix and bed of humans. *Journal of Investigative Dermatology*, 1971, **56**, 61.
6. Samman, P. D. Abnormalities of the finger nails associated with impaired peripheral blood supply. *British Journal of Dermatology*, 1962, **74**, 165.
7. Walters, K. A. Physiochemical characterisation of the human nail: I. pressure sealed apparatus for measuring nail plate permeabilities. *Journal of Investigative Dermatology*, 1981, **7** (2), 76.
8. Zook, E. G. Anatomy and physiology of the perionychium: a review of the literature and anatomic study. *Journal of Hand Surgery*, 1980, **5** (6), 528.

Methods of Observation

Tribal man used keenly attuned and trained senses to survive, but civilised western man has lost much of these natural powers of observation. Thus all health workers need to be retrained to observe curiously, make deductions and formulate hypotheses, testing these by appropriate examinations and procedures.

The fingernails afford an excellent opportunity to practise such observation, as all human beings carry the record of their personality and recent past health in a flat sheet of keratin of the nail plate. Careful examination of the nail plate and the infinite variations in colour, shape and care of the nails may add greatly to overall understanding of the whole person in the clinical or personal examination. Not only are there nearly always signs to observe in even healthy young people (such as habits, mannerisms and manicure), but, increasingly, minor abnormalities in the nutrition or health may have accumulated in the nail plate over recent months. As the thumbnails contain the largest area of nail, they may demonstrate most markedly any lesser changes.

8
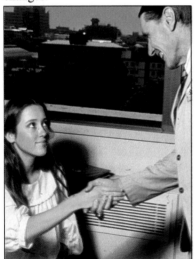
9
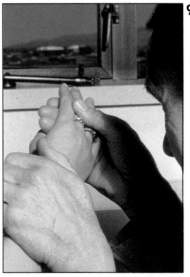

8 The normal approach is to sit down and shake hands whilst having a social chat.

9 The normal two-handed greeting with the examiner's left hand palpating the slightly flexed wrist. The right hand initially holds the fingertips to determine warmth, colour, circulation, etc.

10   The observer now lines up his eye along the line of the nail and the daylight from the window. The normal nail should show a characteristic "shine" from reflected light if held at the proper angle. This angle should be adjusted until a bright light is reflected off the full nail length, thus highlighting abnormalities.

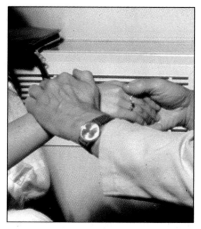

10

Seeing

Have a good light source, preferably sunlight. Light from an angle will reflect off the normally shiny surface of the nail plate. Observing this so-called "shine" on the normal healthy nail is an important part of the proper examination of the fingernails. The fingers and nails may need to be moved up and down until the angle of reflected light is correct, as shown.

In order to be indicative of general disease or disorder, and not due merely to local trauma, changes should be seen in all fingernails of the same hand. Hand-held magnification (usually four or eight times) may be needed, especially where the nails are small.

Feeling

We advocate a fast but careful examination in every person presenting with symptoms of illness. To do this, we suggest "building-in" an examination of the nails to the normal greeting and pulse-taking. In the sequence which follows, in which a natural two-handed greeting leads to the left hand seeking the radial pulse at the wrist, the examiner's right hand may lightly hold the fingers. After observations for *warmth*, *colour* and *shape*, the hand is turned over and the fingers flexed upwards or downwards until the light source reflects on the shiny nail plate. Lastly, the **"springiness"** of the nail pulp over the lunula and the brittleness of the nails are examined.

17

Other Testing Procedures

Unexplained abnormalities on most of the nails should lead to referral to a dermatologist, internist (in general medicine, or the speciality likely to be involved), or podiatrist. These specialists are particularly interested in the nails, their abnormalities and their treatment.

Research procedures such as ultrasound, high-resolution MR imaging, dynamic observations of the capillary blood flow, genetic analysis using DNA probes or determinations of antigens in the nail will become more widely used. Rarely, biopsy of the nail, its bed or surroundings may be advocated by the specialist, and there is now increasing forensic interest in post-mortem examination of nail material.

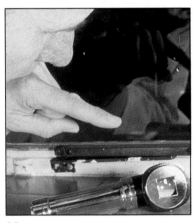

11

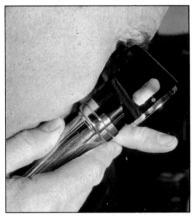

12

11 Method of examination with good sunlight shining down on the nail and the observer standing behind and above. Note also lighted hand lens (lying on table) for closer inspection.
12 Examination of the nail using a lighted magnifying speculum when in poor light.
13 Edge of normal eponychium or proximal nail fold, magnified.

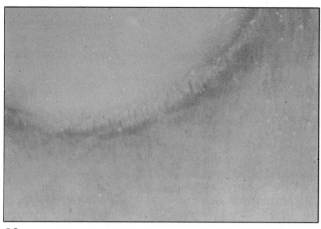

13

References

Blood Flow Techniques

1. Andrade, L. E., Gariel Junior, A., Assad, R. L., Ferrari, A. J. & Atra, E. Panoramic nailfold capillaroscopy: a new reading method and normal range. *Semin. Arthritis. Rheum.,* 1990; **20** (1), 21–31.
2. Arpaia, G., Cimminiello, C., Milani, M., Aloisio, M., Rossi, F., Curri, S. & Bonfardecci, B. A new capillaroscopic assessment of microvascular damage vs Maricq classification in patients with isolated Raynaud phenomenon. *Int. Angiol,* 1989, **8** (3), 129–33.
3. Grassi, W., Felder, M., Thuring-Vollenweider, U. & Bollinger, A. Microvascular dynamics at the nailfold in rheumatoid arthritis. *Clin. Exp. Rheumatol.,* 1989, **7** (1), 47–53.
4. Pazos-Moura, C. C., Moura, E. G., Bouskela, E., Torres, Filho, I. .P. & Breitenbach, M. M. Nailfold capillarscopy in non–insulin-dependent diabetes mellitus; blood flow velocity during rest and post-occlusive reactive hyperaemia. *Clin. Physical.,* 1990, **10** (5), 451–61.

Other Specialised Testing Procedures

1. Bergner, T., Donhauser, G. & Ruzicka, T. Red lunulae in severe alopecia areata. *Acta Dermato-Venereologica,* 1992, **72** (3), 203–5.
2. Holzberg, M. Glomus tumour of the nail. A"red herring" clarified by magnetic resonance imaging. *Archives of Dermatology,* 1992, **128** (2), 160–2.
3. Idy-Peretti, I., Cermakova, E., Dion, E. & Reyagne, P. Subungual glomus tumor: diagnosis based on high-resolution MR images. *American Journal of Roentgenology,* 1992, **159** (6), 1351.

4. Jemec, G. B. & Serup, J. Ultrasound structure of the human nail plate *Arch. Dermatol.,* 1989, **125** (5), 643–6.
5. Kaneshige, T., Takagi, K., Nakamura, S., Hirasawa, T., Sada, M. & Uchida, K. Genetic analysis using fingernail DNA. *Nucleic Acids Research,* 1992, **20** (20), 5489–90.
6. Moriya, F., Miyaishi, S. & Ishizu, H. Presumption of a history of methamphetamine abuse by post-mortem analyses of hair and nails. *Arukoru Kenkyu-To Yakubutsu Ison.* 1992, **27** (2), 152–8.
7. Pierre, M. The Nail. Churchill–Livingstone, Edinburgh, 1981, 3–4.
8. Rich, P. Nail biopsy. Indications and methods. *Journal of Dermatologic Surgery & Oncology,* 1992, **18** (8), 673–82.
9. Scher, R. K. & Ackerman, A. B. Subtle clues to diagnosis from biopsies of nails. The value of nail biopsy for demonstrating fungi not demonstrable by microbiologic techniques. *American Journal of Dermatopathology,* 1980, **2** (1), 55.
10. Stone, O. J., Barr, R. J. & Herten, R. J. Biopsy of the nail area. *Curtis,* 1978, **21** (2), 257.
11. Wegener, R. & Bulnheim, U. Determination of ABO antigens in fingernails using the APAAP (immunoalkalin phosphatase) technique. *Forensic Sci. Int.,* 1990, **46** (1–2), 11–4.

Growth of Nails

The continuous growth from the base of the nail to the free edge is rapid in small children (6–8 weeks), but in normal adults varies between 0.5 and 1.2 mm/week and about 4–6 months in the "young" elderly. Nail plate growth thus slows 25–33% over a normal lifetime.

Because steady growth occurs each day, a few days of serious illness give rise to that most helpful of clinical signs in the nails: the growth arrest line (see discussion under the heading "Beau's Lines", Chapter 2). William Bean measured his own left thumbnail growth each day over 30 years, and found this to be 0.123 mm/day at 32 years of age and 0.100 mm/day when aged 61.

Temperature probably has some effect, as earlier polar observations showed slowed growth rates, but evidence of this remains controversial.

As the nails grow faster on longer fingers, the fastest growth occurs in the middle finger, followed by the ring and index fingers. Hamilton *et al.* (1955) in their classic study showed that growth rate was most significantly related to ageing. Whilst the nails grew more slowly in later decades, they were thicker. Thus, in old people with normal digital blood supply, the same unit mass of nail is probably formed each day.

More recently, studies by Griffiths & Reshad (1983) have confirmed the previous observations that trauma stimulates growth. The nails of the right hand grow faster in right-handed people, as the dominant hand is used more often and is thus subjected to more minor trauma.

Dawber (1981) also confirmed that immobility can slow up the rate of nail growth. Some rare and unusual conditions, such as the yellow nail syndrome described by Samman (1986), also lead to very slow growth. The reason that slowed growth occurs in paralysed fingers has not been explained, but is due probably to nerve effects on capillary blood flow.

In middle life it takes 3–4 months for the fingernail to grow from proximal matrix cells to the free edge. Knowing this, one can identify the approximate time frame of a generalised serious illness of more than a few days by the position of a transverse growth arrest line (Beau's line). Small white spots—the result of minor and often insignificant trauma—can also be a useful marker of nutritional normality as illustrated. As would be expected, older, more slowly growing nails become thicker, but this may also be due to transonychial water loss.

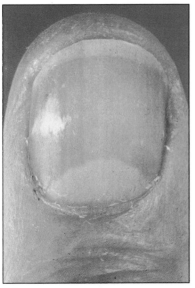 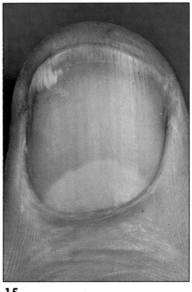

14

15

14 1st photograph of thumb.
15 2nd photograph 6 weeks later. Nail growth in a 58-year-old physician over 6 weeks as measured by movement of "white spot" resulting from previous injury.

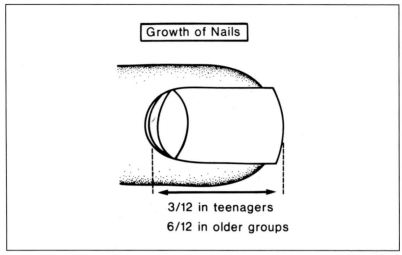

16

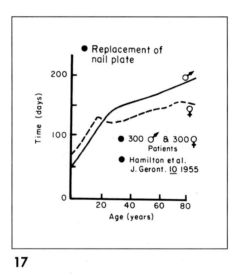

17

16   Diagram showing average growth of nails for different age groups.

17   Approximate guide to growth rates; 6–8 months for full regrowth would be seen in 70-year-olds.

18 & 19   Fast and slow nail growth.

```
┌─────────────────────────────────────┐
│  SLOW NAIL GROWTH                   │
│                                     │
│   ● Age                             │
│   ● Genetic                         │
│   ● ♀s                              │
│                                     │
│   not: hair                         │
│         baldness                    │
│         fat                         │
│         height & weight             │
└─────────────────────────────────────┘
```
18

```
┌─────────────────────────────────────┐
│  FAST NAIL GROWTH                   │
│                                     │
│   ● Nail biting                     │
│   ● Damage nail tip                 │
│   ● 1st finger                      │
└─────────────────────────────────────┘
```
19

References

1. Baran, R. Nail growth direction revisited. Why do nails grow out instead of up? *Journal of the American Academy of Dermatology,* 1981, **4** (1), 78.

2. Bean, W. B. Nail growth 10 years of observation. *Archives of Internal Medicine,* 1974, **134**, 479.

3. Dawber, R. The effect of immobilization on fingernail growth. *Clinical and Experimental Dermatology,* 1981, **6** (5), 533.

4. Donovan, K. M. Antarctic environment and nail growth. *British Journal of Dermatology,* 1977, **96** (5), 507.

5. Griffiths, W. A. & Reshad, H. Hair and nail growth: an investigation of the role of left and right handedness. *Clinical and Experimental Dermatology,*1983, **8** (2), 129.

6. Hamilton, J. B., Terada, H. & Mestler, G. E. Studies of growth throughout the lifespan in Japanese; growth and size of nails and their relationship to age, sex, heredity and other factors. *Journal of Gerontology,* 1955, **10**, 401.

7. Jemec, G. B., Agner, T. & Serup, J. Transonychial water loss: relation to sex, age and nail–plate thickness. *British Journal of Dermatology,* 1989, **121** (4), 443–6.

Infant Nails

Seaborg and Bodurtha (1992) carefully examined and took the pregnancy history associated with 48 newly born infants. They found fingernails more useful than toenails because at birth the latter are too small and there is, for an unknown reason, greater variation in toenails.

In Infants:
- Nail size did not vary between sexes.
- Possibly, first fingernails are longer in Caucasian than Afro-American babies.
- At full term, nails in fingers reach the end of the fingertips, but toenails do not.
- A curved impression on the fingertip edge or distal groove is a remnant of an embryological structure and "grows out".
- Fingernails and toenails should all resemble each other, but fingernails and toenails are not the same shape.
- More than a quarter of infants with "foetal alcohol syndrome" or whose mothers have misused drugs have nail dysplasias.
- Maternal drugs such as phenytoin may cause dysplasias (1–2%).
- Ectodermal dysplasias, Trisomy 18, nail-patella syndromes and other congenital disorders may be suspected because of nail dysplasias in the newborn child.

The nail is expected to be somewhat soft and fragile in the newborn. There are as yet few reports on normal nail developments between 24 and 32 weeks *in utero*.

References

1. Ballard, J. L., Novak, K. K. & Driver, M. A simplified score for assessment of foetal maturation of newly born infants. *Journal of Pediatrics,* 1979, **95**, 769–74.
2. Crain, L. S., Fitzmaurice, N. E. & Mondry, C. Nail dysplasia and fetal alcohol syndrome *Am. J. Dis. Child,* 1983, **137**, 1069–72.
3. Ernhart, C. B., Wolf, A. W., Linn, P. L., *et al.* Alcohol-related birth defects: Syndromal anomalies, intra-uterine growth retardation, and neonatal behavioural assessment. *Alcoholism,* 1985, **9**, 447–53.
4. Hudson, V. K., Flannery, D. B., Karp, W. B., *et al.* Finger and nail measurements in newborn infants. *Dysmorphol. Clin. Genet. ,*1988, **1**,145–7.
5. Seaborg & Bodurtha, J. Nail size in normal infants. *Clinical Pediatrics.* 1992, **28**, 142–145.
6. Zalas, N. Embryology of the human nail. *Arch. Dermatol.,* 1963, **87**, 37–53.

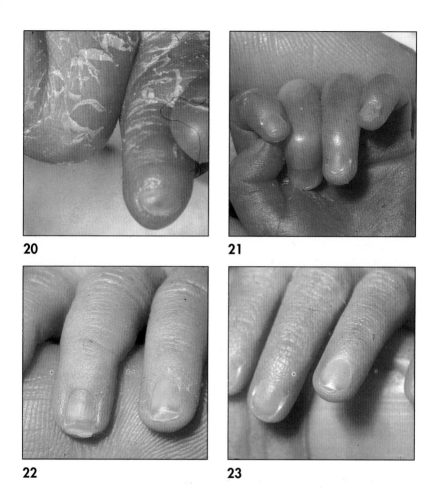

20 Nails from a 27-week premature infant. Note normal nail development (lowest nail), abnormal nail and syndactyly (top of picture).

21 The 30–32-week appearance of otherwise normal neonate. Note immaturity also of skin.

22 Full-term infant from abnormal pregnancy (blood pressure treatment). Note brown lines near the free edge of all fingers, suggesting lysis index.

23 Full-term infant nails from normal pregnancy.

Normal Nail Appearances

Normal people in normal health and with normal nutrition have normal-looking nails with only minor variations.

The specialised matrix cells can react in only relatively few ways if blood supply or nutrition is impaired over a period of time. Such insults grow out to the free edge and are visible for several months. More distal changes can, however, be the result of bacterial or finger infections ascending under the nail in persons with reduced local or general immunity. Insufficient scientific studies have been carried out on large enough groups of subjects to ascertain whether dietary factors may influence texture and appearance. Studies on flexibility and hardness of the nails (Ramrakhiani, 1978; Finlay *et al.* 1980) have also reported that detergents, organic chemicals, oils, etc. may be factors in the occupational environment which affects the nail plate. A group of people in various occupations are presented to describe the wide limits of normality found in those who were otherwise in good general health.

In the general examination of the patient, we believe that signs of occupational activity may allow the examiner to establish a quicker rapport than would otherwise be the case. There is a need to be aware of the responsibility of employer and employee in such cases, as in many countries the documentation of such appearances may be of greater importance in industrial compensation and legal procedures.

24 Normal first or index fingernail in a young woman.
25 Normal nail of a young woman in her 20's.
26 Normal thumbnail with a hint of Beau's lines in a 27-year-old female scientific officer.
27 Normal thumbnail of a young female laboratory assistant.

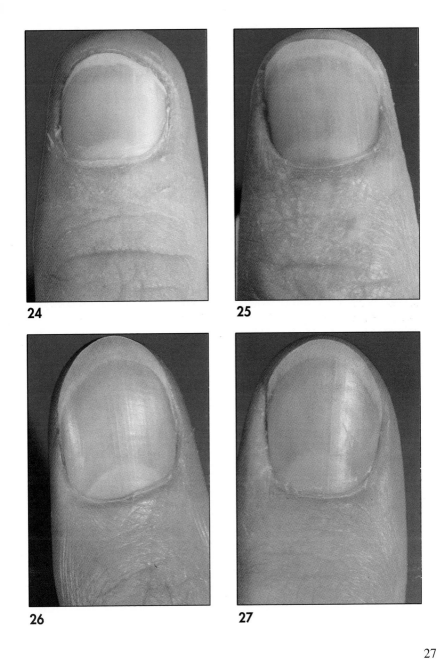

24

25

26

27

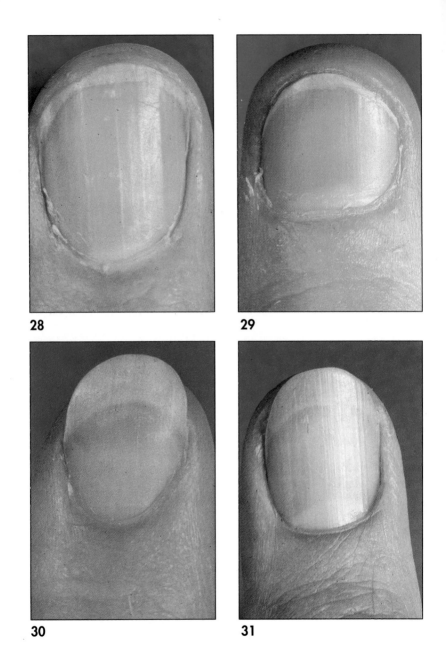

28

29

30

31

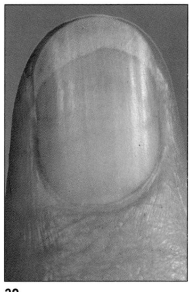
32

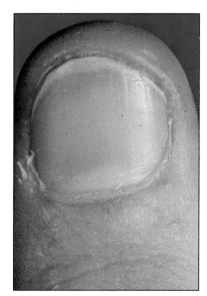
33

28 Normal thumbnail of a young female laboratory assistant.
29 Normal nails of young female clerical assistant.
30 Normal thumbnail from a healthy female laboratory worker in her 20s.
31 Normal thumbnail of a young female laboratory assistant.
32 Normal thumbnail of a 22-year-old laboratory technician.
33 Normal thumbnail of a healthy female laboratory worker in her 20s.

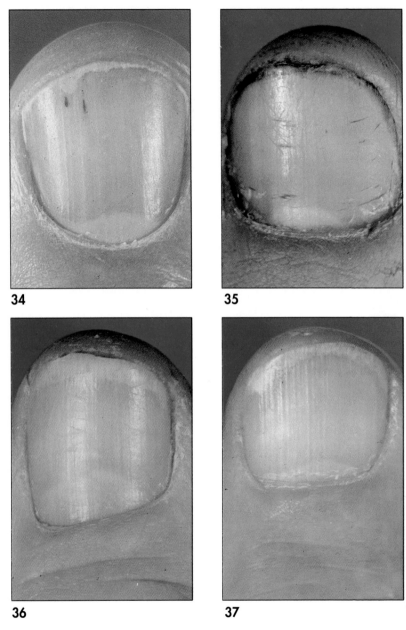

34

35

36

37

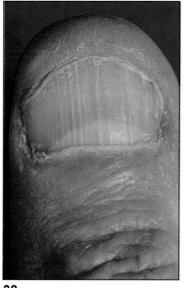

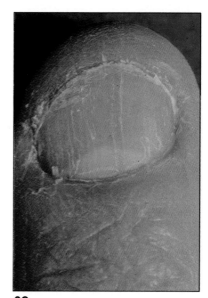

38　　　　　　　　　　　**39**

34　Normal thumbnail of young fitter and turner. The two "splinter" haemorrhages and localised onycholysis are due to local trauma.

35　Normal thumbnail of a motor mechanic. Note the ingrained oil and occupational scratches on the nail plate.

36　Normal thumbnail of a healthy 40-year-old electrician. Note the minor occupational changes in the nail.

37　Thumbnail of hospital house manager. Note small white spots on the free edge dating from minor trauma 3 months ago. Longitudinal ridges are a normal variation in middle life.

38　Normal thumbnail from a 62-year-old woman whose life-long hobby is working in her rock garden. Nails show occupational changes typical of rough and active hard use.

39　Normal thumbnail of a young female employed as a washing-up assistant in a laboratory.

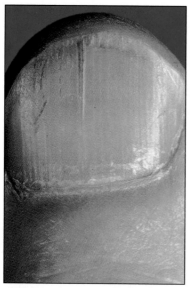

40

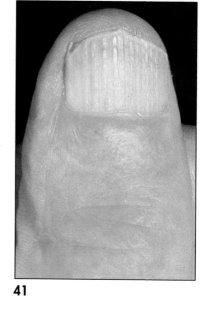

41

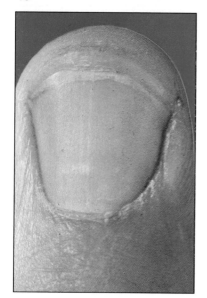

42

40 Normal thumbnail of a male laboratory worker. Note the abnormal single longitudinal ridge.

41 Nail of retired post office worker, 72 years of age, said to be in good health. However, he has rather opaque nails with beading. Nutritional changes may be related to alcohol use. The opacity and broken ridges are abnormal findings in a person of this age.

42 Fingernail of a guitar-player. Note the very short and typically thick pad of flesh over the tip of the finger.

References

1. Cohen, P. H. & Scher, R. K. Nail disease and dermatology *J. Am. Dermatol.,* 1989, **21** (5 Pt 1), 1020–2.
2. Finlay, A.Y., Frost, P., Keith, A. D. & Snipes, W. An assessment of factors influencing flexibility of human fingernails. *British Journal of Dermatology,*1980, **103** (4), 357.
3. Forslind, B., Nordstrom, G., Toijer, D. & Eriksson, K. The rigidity of human fingernails: a biophysical investigation on influencing physical parameters. *Acta Dermato-Venereologica* (Stockholm)*,* 1980, **60** (3), 217.
4. Jarrett, A. & Spearman, R. I. C. Histochemistry of the human nail. *Archives of Dermatology,* 1966, **94**, 652.
5. Ramrakhiani, M. Indentation and hardness studies of human nails. *Indian Journal of Biochemistry and Biophysics,* 1978, **15** (4), 341.
6. Samman, P. D. & Fenton, D. A. *The Nails in Disease.* Heinemann, London, 1986.

Minor Variations from Normal

Because of the slower rate of forward growth, thickening of the nail normally occurs with increasing age, and longitudinal ridges appear on the surface. Normally, such longitudinal ridges seldom occur before the age of 40 years and, when present, may suggest an associated chromosomal or congenital defect.

More increased curving (convex or concave) in such disorders as clubbing, koilonychia, etc. is always associated with a more generalised systemic disorder until a careful clinical search and analysis of tests on blood and nail clippings have eliminated abnormality.

We have repeatedly noticed minor variations of the nails present in people with other general chronic medical illnesses. These have been included in the appropriate sections. Marked longitudinal ridging, beading of the ridges and pitting of the nail plate do not occur in normal, young, healthy subjects. These appearances would suggest a more biochemical or medical search for otherwise unsuspected illness.

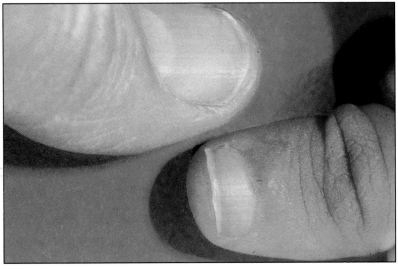

43

43 Small nail. Micronychia in intellectually impaired patient. (Normal control nail above.)

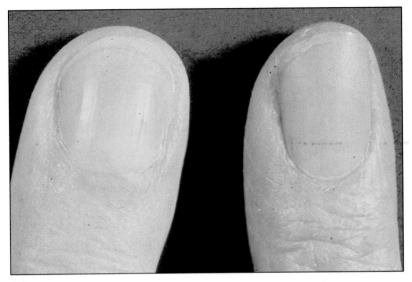

44

44 Variation in width. A normal variation in width and curvature seen in the left finger and not associated with any illness or known disease.

45 Triangular lunula. The triangular lunula in the thumb of an obsessive female filing clerk; the nail base, growth arrest lines and white streak suggest excessive manicure.

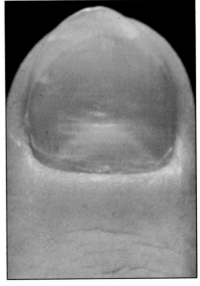

45

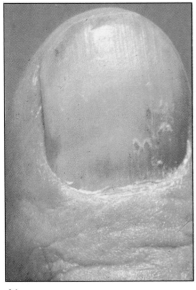
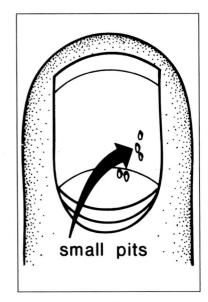

small pits

46

46   Small pits. These greenish coloured nails show bands of pigment but the example shown here illustrates pitting. Pitting of the nails is sometimes called Rosenau's Depressions. Psoriasis has been excluded. When widespread may produce so-called "thimble-nail".

47   Minor pitting in well-kept nails of a 29-year-old shop assistant. Search well for "hidden" psoriasis on elbows, knees or scalp! (Not found here, however.)

48   Marked beading in an elderly and somewhat socially neglected pensioner with thyroxicosis.

49   Beading. Beading present in the longitudinal ridges of a middle-aged woman with poor manicure. Short nail may suggest some trisomy, and lack of lunula also sometimes congenital. Patient appeared of normal intelligence with no serious systemic disease.

50   Marked "beading" on fingernail. Hypothyroid male on treatment with thyroxine for hypothyroidism. Note lack of beading near lunula and failure of care, strongly suggesting lapse in treatment medication.

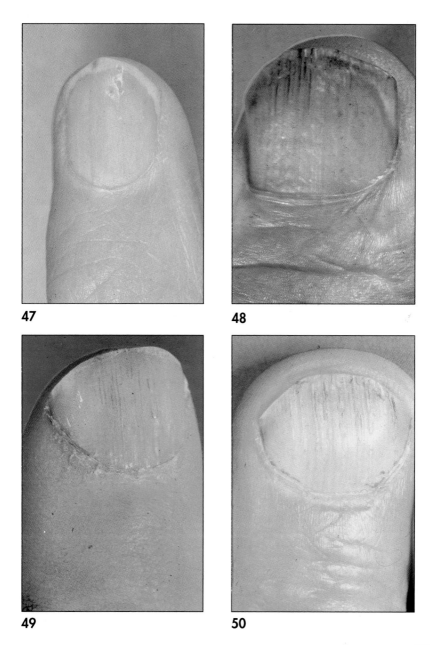

47

48

49

50

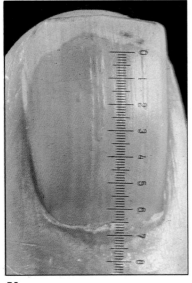 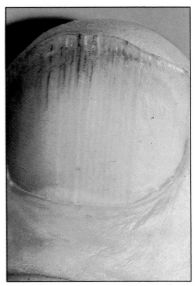

51   **52**

51   Measurement of beading. Fifth finger on the left hand of a small woman, showing marked beading. Actual mm scale shows "bead" to be 0.2–0.3 mm in length.

52   Ridges. Longitudinal ridges in a man with chronic obstructive airways disease and mild hypoxaemia ($pAO_2=70$).

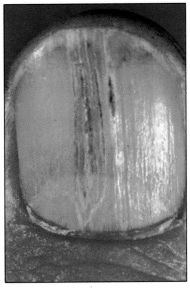
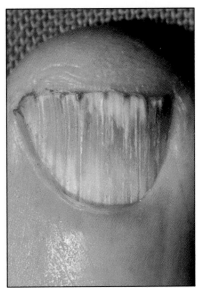

53   **54**

53 Very marked ridging. Longitudinal ridges in an elderly man with renal failure. Note that "pigment" in ridge is dirt from his hobby of rose gardening.

54 Brachyonychia. Normal variation of short nail or brachyonychia. So-called "racquet nail". Sometimes seen with other congenital abnormalities. Look for toe changes, alterations in facial bones (Rubenstein & Taylor, 1963) and, occasionally, septal defects. Note also very marked and abnormal ridging and pigment band. These changes could be regarded as senile in many elderly patients, but the illustration is of a man in his late 20s.

Changes Related to Care, Occupation, Personality & Brittleness

In 20th century human beings, the immediate environment, both internal and external, remains hostile, but well-adjusted urbanised or town-dwelling individuals with personal security and confidence, and who remain in good health with a stable personality, should have well-kept and well-groomed nails.

Personality traits may be revealed in nail or cuticle biting. These and other habit tics may result in short, abnormally thickened nail plates, ridging and opacity. The cuticle may be pulled back from the nail, and indeed, over-zealous manicure may leave a site for entry of local or foreign bacteria or fungi. Occupational activity giving rise to thickened, pitted, opaque or shiny, smooth nails should be revealed by history taking.

Occasionally, paronychia or fungal infections result from over-zealous manicure of the cuticle. This or nail-biting may result in shredding of the proximal nail fold. This is also called "hang nail". Unexplained transverse ridging found only on one nail may be caused by cuticle pressure from orange sticks or teeth.

References

1. Barnett, J. M. & Scher, R. K. Nail cosmetics. *International Journal of Dermatology,* 1992, **31** (10), 675–81.
2. Baran, R. Nail biting and picking as a possible cause of longitudinal melanonychia. A study of 6 cases. *Dermatologica,* 1990, **181** (2), 126–8.
3. Bhatia, V. N, Possible multiplication of *M. leprae* on skin and nail bed of a laboratory worker. *Indian Journal of Leprosy.,* 1990, **62** (2), 226–7.
4. Calnan, C. D. Reactions to artificial colouring materials, *Journal of the Society of Cosmetic Chemistry,* 1967, **18**, 215.
5. Fisher, A. A. Permanent loss of fingernails due to allergic reaction to an acrylic nail preparation: a sixteen-year follow-up study. *Cutis,* 1989, **43** (5), 404–6.
6. London, L., Jourbert, G., Manjra, S. I., Krause, L. B, Dermatoses – anoccupational hazard in the canning industry. *South African Medical Journal* 1992, **81** (12), 606–12.
7. Rayan, G. M., Turner, W. T. Hand complications in children from digital sucking. *Journal of Hand Surgery,* 1989, **14** (6), 933–6.
8. Samman, P.D. Onychia due to synthetic nail coverings. Experimental studies, *Transactions of the St John's Hospital,* Dermatological Society, London, 1961, **46**, 68.
9. Samman, P. D. A traumatic nail dystrophy produced by a habit tic. *Archives of Dermatology,* 1963, **88**, 895.
10. Samman, P. D. Nail disorders caused by external influences. *Journal of the Society of Cosmetic Chemistry,* 1977, **28**, 351.

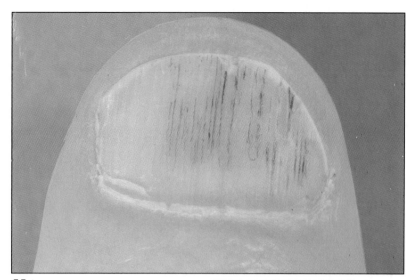

55

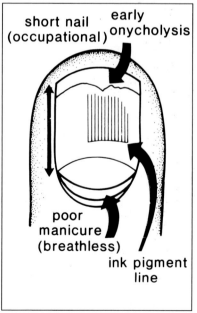

short nail (occupational) early onycholysis

poor manicure (breathless)

ink pigment line

55 An example of onychorrhexis (*see Glossary, Chapter 16*). Many abnormalities manifest in the nails of this 64-year-old printing operator with chronic obstructive airways disease and autoimmune hypothyroidism. He has not worked for 6 weeks, but note the pigment (ink) line in the nails. He is being treated with thyroxine. Note also poor manicure.

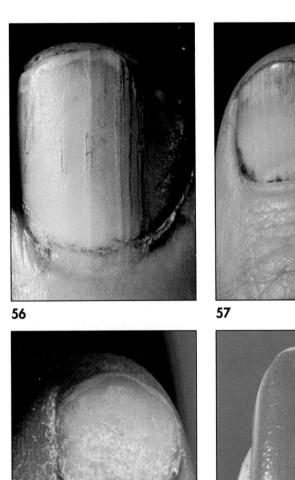

56

57

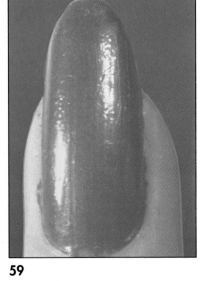

58

59

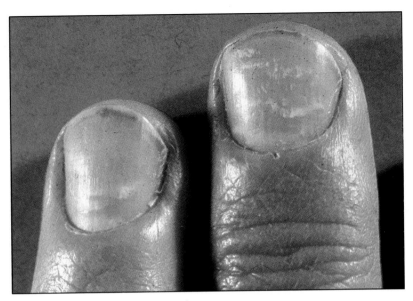

60

56   Poor manicure: Why? Poor manicure as an indication of mental depression. The nail of a depressed widower in his late 60's. Note prominent longitudinal ridges.

57   Poor manicure. Poor trimming and cutting of nails with poor manicure in motor car garage labourer.

58   Chemical damage. Dystrophy in a 36-year-old barman. This is most likely due to chemical damage from detergent powder used for washing glasses in a small area of contact. Possibly also a nutritional element from excessive intake of "empty" alcohol calories.

59   Camouflage. Normal nail, possibly slightly curved, of a hospital receptionist. Very well disguised! Danger of onycholysis.

60   *Leukonychia striata.* Excessive manicure and pushing down of "quick" leads to white transverse injury lines—similar to *Leukonychia striata.* When such variations are seen on all nails, this could be described as *L. variegata.*

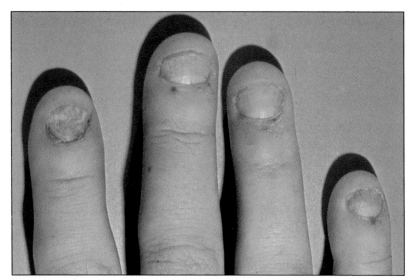

61

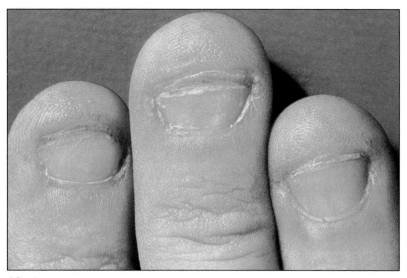

62

44

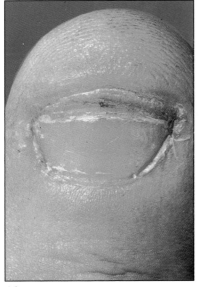

63

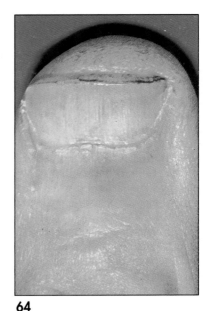

64

61 Nails of distressed housewife. Example of evidence of background and general medical conditions from various changes in the nails on one hand. Note filling in of nail fold due to mild bronchiectasis. Also paronychia of index fingernail, suggesting immersion in water due to washing dishes or clothes.

62 Nail biting of all fingers. Brachyonchia or "short" nail has resulted in the middle finger.

63 Damage from nail biting. Close-up of the same fingernail on the hands of an anxious clerk.

64 Personality difficulties? Nail-bitten finger of a 55-year-old, rather simple driver, who lost his job through heavy drinking. Note short nail, lack of care and pigment.

65 Habit "tic". Central damage to right thumb due to life-long habit "tic". Nail scratched on right upper canine tooth under stress.

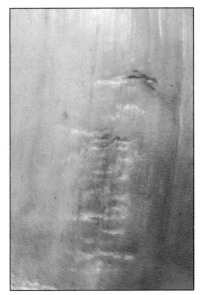

65

Brittle, Breakable & Fragile Nails

Brittle, fragile and easily breakable nails are a common presentation to family physicians. They are usually due to a rapid change in the water content of the nail plate or a change in the content and make-up of the keratin plate, so that any general disorder which causes a change in blood supply, nerve impulses and control of terminal plexus of vessels, or changes in the content of nutrients, will lead to brittle nails. A distinction has sometimes been made between the different forms of nail splitting which occur in various forms of brittle nails, such as lamellar splitting of the free edge, transverse splitting near the distal margin, or the isolated split extending proximally.

In general medical practice, one excludes any other skin disease, identifies general medical conditions and moves to measure nutrients and hormonal status. In some troublesome cases (mainly in housewives), occupational causes can be countered by wearing rubber gloves. The nail content of sulphur-containing amino acids and minerals is occasionally helpful in diagnosis.

The most common causes of brittle nails are:

1. *Exposure to local chemical substances*
- Excess water.
- Alkalis.
- Excessive detergents.
- Oils used in garages and industry.
- Solvents.
- Oxidising agents, etc.

2. *General skin disorders*
- Psoriasis.
- Lichen planus.

3. *General medical disorders*
- Thyroid disease or lack of growth hormone.
- Chronic heart failure (usually coronary disease or failed hypertensive).
- Peripheral ischaemia with atheroma of the aortic arch.
- Elderly malnutrition (check sulphur-containing amino acids, thiamin in blood, vitamin C in white cells).
- Chronic blood loss—where associated with koilonychia.

4. *Neurological disorders*
- Such as hemiparesis and peripheral neuropathies (especially alcohol).

References

1. Kechijian, P. Brittle Fingernails. *Dermatol. Clin.*, 1985, **3**, 421–9.
2. Lubach, D. & Beckers, P. Wet working conditions increase brittleness of nails, but do not cause it. *Dermatology*, 1992, **185** (2), 120–2.

Chapter 2

Transverse Growth Arrest Lines ("Beau's Lines")

Transverse lines or depressions right across most of the nails as a result of previous illness are called Beau's lines (1846). These are important because they can be seen easily in the standard observation of nails which follows the normal introduction and hand shaking.

If due to significant illness, the lines will be seen on all nails on one or both hands. Although no definitivet documentation exists, common observation indicates that a serious febrile illness lasting several days, or a less serious metabolic upset for a week or so, is required to produce such lines. Sudden, very severe, short episodes of illness, for example, a life-threatening haemorrhage with hypotension, can produce such discernible transverse ridges across all nails.

The value of the observation lies in a standard examination of the nail in all subjects. Knowing that the growth rate from base to free edge is about 3 months in a young adult and about 4–6 months in an elderly person assists in dating one or more episodes of illness and concurrent growth arrest. It should be noted that in chronic ill health, arterial insufficiency or inadequate states of nutrition, the growth rate of the nail may be slower. This occurs especially in the toenails of elderly men with arterial insufficiency. Here, metabolic or growth arrest lines can take up to 8 or 12 months to grow out to the free edge.

Should the duration of the illness or drug reaction be of sufficient severity for more than one week, the transverse line or depression may lead to a total division of the nail plate, referred to as "onychomadesis". This will grow slowly outwards before the distal part is shed at the free end of the nail.

As well as in cases of severe metabolic illness, which may include such disorders as measles in childhood, zinc deficiency or Stevens–Johnson syndrome, Beau's lines are also seen in many drug reactions involving the skin and when cytotoxic agents are used. Usually, all nails are involved, but when only one or two fingernails or toenails are affected, local pressures, traumas or chronic eczematous conditions can be found.

Some studies suggest that the use of polarised light may be helpful in examining fingernail ridges. In order to see such growth arrest lines easily, the fingernails must be held at the correct angle to the on-coming light. The transverse ridges will then be highlighted across the normal shine of the nails.

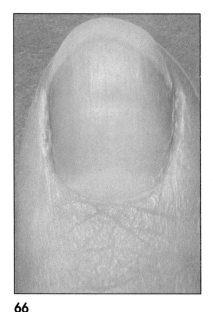

66

66 Single Beau's line. Beau's line in a young woman with post-operative complications some 2 months previously.

67 & 68 Slightly differing views of same finger showing growth arrest line.

69 Recurrent illness. Thumbnail of a 28-year-old hotel receptionist with bronchial asthma. Intermittent high steroid dosage has led to a series of growth arrest lines (Beau's lines).

70 Beau's from the side. Two severe growth arrest lines in a 34-year-old female with sub-acute bacterial endocarditis, initially partly treated. Note early "filling" in of nail fold but no definite clubbing.

71 Evidence of two illnesses. Two growth arrest lines in a nurse who experienced a severe bleeding episode and splenectomy 6 weeks later.

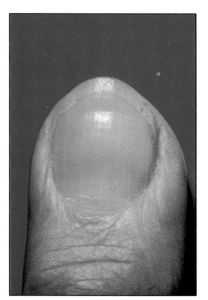

67

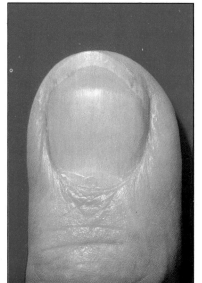

68

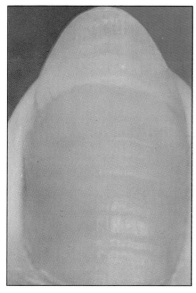

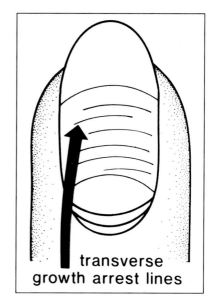

transverse
growth arrest lines

69

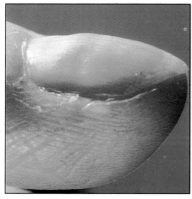

70

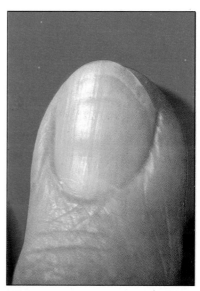

71

49

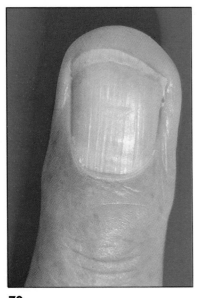

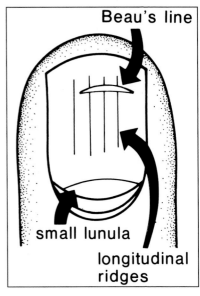

72

73

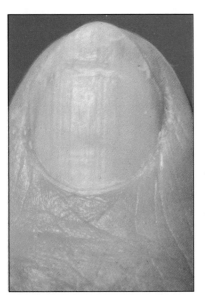

72 With other signs. A 72-year-old hypertensive woman with serum albumen 3.2 g/l and poor nutritional habits. A minor myocardial infarction about 5 months previously resulted in Beau's lines on all nails.

73 Variations in lines. Beau's lines on the nail of a young secretary experiencing repeated attacks of asthma. Note marked growth arrest line near tip of nail and minimal lines near the lunula.

74 Severe illness. Severe growth arrest for 3 months in an elderly woman who was severely ill during this period of time after post-operative and successful bowel cancer resection.

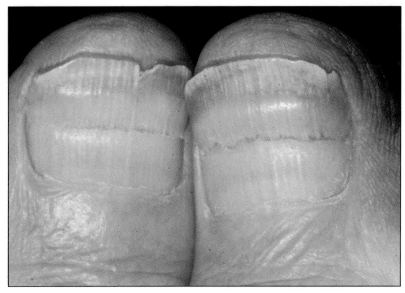

74

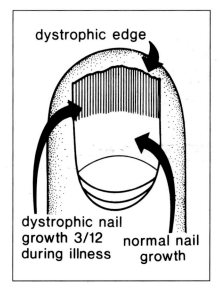

dystrophic edge

dystrophic nail
growth 3/12
during illness

normal nail
growth

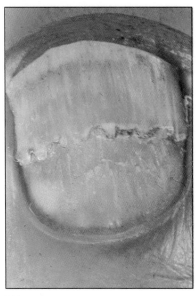

75 Complete growth arrest. Complete and severe arrest line. Major and severe life-threatening illness 6 weeks previously.

75

References

1. Apolinar, E. & Rowe, W. F. Examination of human fingernail ridges by means of polarized light. *Journal of Forensic Science,* 1980, **25** (1), 154.
2. Beau, J. H. S. Certain caracteres de semeliologie retrospective, presentes par les ongles. *Archives in General Medicine,* 1946, **9**, 447.
3. Kitahara, T. & Ogawa, H. Cultured nail keratinocytes express hard keratins characteristic of nail and hair *in vivo. Archives of Dermatological Research,* 1992, **284** (4), 253–6.
4. Mishra, D., Singh, G. & Pandey, S. S. Possible carbamaz-epine–induced reversible onychomadesis. *International Journal of Dermatology,* 1989, **28** (7), 460–1.
5. Patki, A. H. & Mehta, J. M. Dapsone-induced erythroderma with Beau's lines. *Lepr. Rev.,* 1989, **60** (4), 274–7.
6. Ward, J. A. *Clinical Methods,* Hurst, J. W. (ed), Butterworth, Boston, 1981, 542.
7. Weismann, K. Lines of Beau: possible markers of zinc deficiency. *Acta Dermato-Venereologica* (Stockholm), 1977, **57** (1), 88.

Chapter 3
Koilonychia or Spoon Nails

The maximal growth of the matrix cells is in the centre of the nail to give the normal curvature. However, as in many deficiency states the blood supply is good to each side of the nail, the cells grow satisfactorily whilst the centre remains flattened. Eventually, the flattening becomes a hollow or even "spoon-shaped". This descriptive term is derived from the Greek word '*koilos*' or spoon.

In the early stages of koilonychia, the nail becomes increasingly flattened, later developing a true concavity. The nail surface is often smoother than normal, especially in early koilonychia. As there are many causes of koilonychia (*see Table 1*), the thickness of the nail plate is a reflection of the underlying disorder. Thus, koilonychia associated with iron deficiency usually shows softer and thinner nails. The thinness may, however, be due to the associated poor nutritional status and poor intake of sulphur-containing amino acids.

The normal keratin plate of the nails is formed by the incorporation of sulphur-containing amino acids into the cells. To do this, amino acid transport across the cell membrane must be normal. Insulin and growth hormone must be present in permissive amounts to allow such transport. Thus, people with diabetes and less than adequate amounts of circulating insulin (i.e. "poorly controlled" diabetics), with mean daily blood glucose values two or three times above normal, may show flattening of the nails and, later, koilonychia. In such koilonychia, other nail dystrophy, such as thickening, is common because of slowed growth. There have been suggestions based on observations of Ladakhis that genetic and seasonal influences are both important when koilonychia is widespread (*see References*).

The active matrix or nail-forming cells demand high levels of iron and copper for their metallo-enzymes. Koilonychia can thus be found in:
- Iron deficiency anaemia.
- Reduction in total body iron.
- Low iron stores without severe anaemia.

Since several biochemical steps are required to form normal nail, a genetic failure at any one of these stages may result in koilonychia. The nail-patella syndrome is one such rare example.

As the returning arterioles from the digital pulp plexus enter the nail matrix from each side, this suggests that deficiencies in nail formation, as well as flattening, may well be seen centrally in the first instance (*see Figure 84*). This hypothesis is at least as convincing as that put forward by

Stone (1967), who suggests that koilonychia is a change of angulation of the principal matrix secondary to connective tissue changes. He suggests that spooning will occur if the distal end of the matrix is relatively low compared with the proximal end.

Concerning flattened nails and koilonychia, it is most essential to ascertain whether the condition has always been present. In some families, or in famine areas (such as the Horn of Africa), growth hormone demand in early life may give rise to some koilonychia, as there is insufficient growth hormone for both bones and cell membrane transport sites. This should disappear after primary school age if nutrition is adequate.

Because of the variety of possible underlying causes and the commonness of minor degrees of this condition, its importance as a diagnostic sign is often overlooked—hence the wide range of examples. Koilonychia may also be secondary to occupational hazards (such as solvents), local injury or psoriasis, or in association with Raynaud's phenomenon. If koilonychia is not due to occupational disease or local skin conditions (excluded by careful search), then over 90% of people seen in general practice or internal medicine have either iron deficiency, an inadequate intake of essential sulphur-containing amino acids or long-term diabetes mellitus. (For a further treatment of nail changes resulting from diabetes, see Chapter 11.)

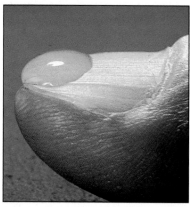

76

76 Early koilonychia. "Drop of water test": an old-fashioned but once popular test for spooning of nails. General appearance and normality of nail are more useful signs in early koilonychia.

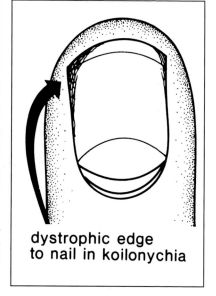

dystrophic edge to nail in koilonychia

TABLE 1. *Causes of Koilonychia*

SULPHUR IN THUMBNAILS

- **Controls**

7 papers	= 3.15%	1914–1937 (2.7–3.8)

- **ChCh Controls**

  = 3.24%   (3.2–3.34)

- **Diabetics**

  = 2.9%   (2.1–3.2)

  SIG diff .01

CYSTEINE IN NAILS %

- **Up to 1933** — 5 papers
- **Normals** — 11.1% (8.8–13.5)
- **Diabetics** — 8.7% (6) (6.3–9.8)

  SIG .01 level

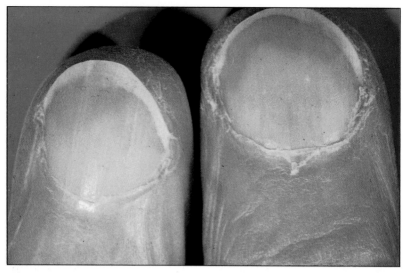

77

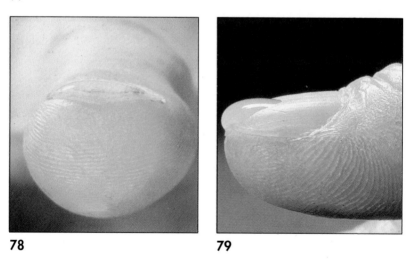

78

79

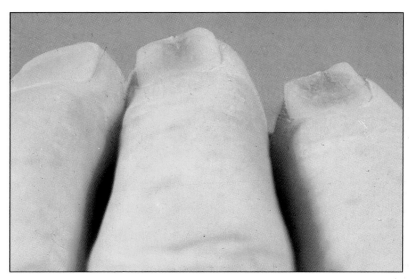

80

77   Koilonychia as part of deficiency state. Thin, flat nails in a 67-year-old woman with anaemia due to nutritional deficiency (documented low albumen, iron and folate). Note also loss of lunula and poor manicure, suggesting loss of interest in personal state.

78   Koilonychia in diabetes. Koilonychia—diabetic nail with high blood sugars, raised growth hormone and nail dystrophy in a male aged 37.

79   Drop of water test. Water test for koilonychia.

80   Koilonychia—nail variation. Dorsal view of hand with koilonychia showing marked variation in degree of flattening or spooning in different nails.

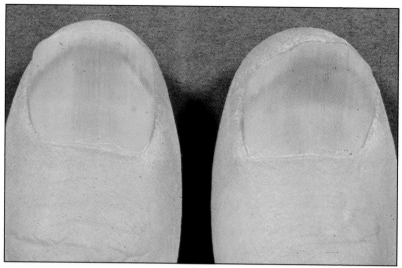

81

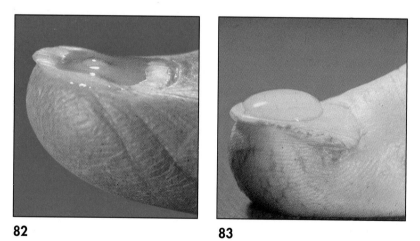

82　　　　　　　　　　　**83**

81　Koilonychia and thin nails. Koilonychia—fingers of an older woman with combined anaemia and nutritional deficiency.

82　Combined deficiency. Severe spooning with some thinning of the nail in a 72-year-old depressed woman with combined deficiency of iron and protein intake.

83　Free edge dystrophy. Although the thumb or great toe (1st toe) has the largest volume of nail and thus shows maximal changes, other nails also show changes.

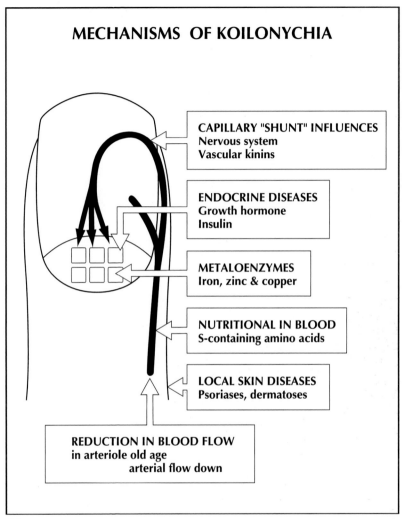

MECHANISMS OF KOILONYCHIA

CAPILLARY "SHUNT" INFLUENCES
Nervous system
Vascular kinins

ENDOCRINE DISEASES
Growth hormone
Insulin

METALOENZYMES
Iron, zinc & copper

NUTRITIONAL IN BLOOD
S-containing amino acids

LOCAL SKIN DISEASES
Psoriases, dermatoses

REDUCTION IN BLOOD FLOW
in arteriole old age
arterial flow down

84

84 A semi-diagrammatic schema showing the multiple mechanisms which may produce koilonychia of the severity seen in **82** & **83**.

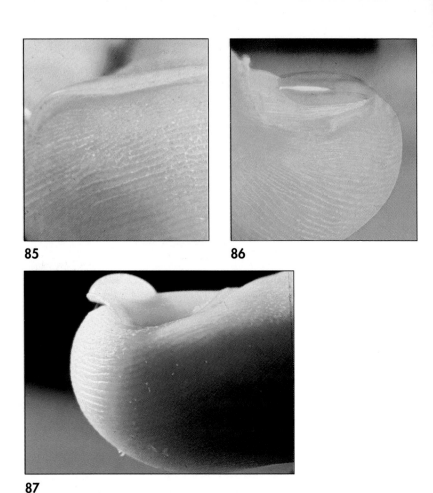

85 Insulin-deficient koilonychia. Marked nail dystrophy and koilonychia in a middle-aged male diabetic. Serum and bone marrow iron were normal, but there was moderately severe insulin deficiency over 10–15 years.

86 Koilos in short thumbnail. Koilonychia—same 37-year-old male diabetic. Note thickness of dystrophic nail in clerical worker. Due to excess sugar and growth hormone?

87 Raised free edge. "Drop of water" test for koilonychia.

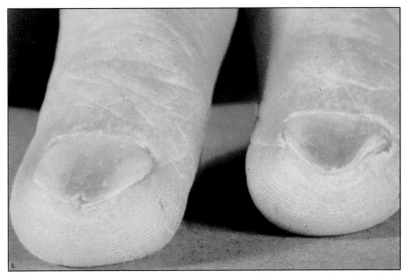

88

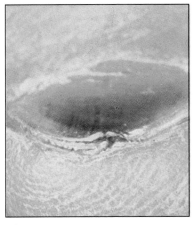

89

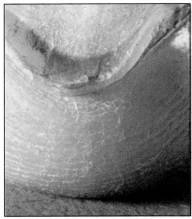

90

88 Severe classical koilonychia. Severe long-term iron deficiency resulting in gross koilonychia in a 60-year-old woman of reduced intelligence.

89 Koilonychia, pigment and nail splitting. Severe koilonychia with pigmentation and splitting of the nail's free edge.

90 Dramatic spooning. Close-up of free edge of nail to show dramatic "spooning" and thickening in koilonychia.

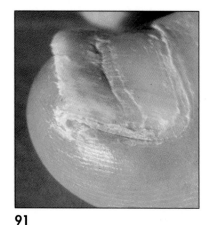

91

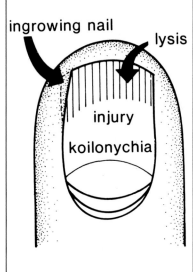

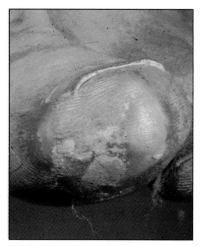

92

91 Multiple signs in toe. Great toenails also show the koilonychia seen best in the thumb nails. Note also old injury, paronychia and poor manicure.

92 Diabetic toe koilonychia. Severe koilonychia B in a middle-aged diabetic man with normal serum iron and no anaemia. Note damage to toe pulp.

References

1. Anand, I. S. & Harris, P. Koilonychia in Ladakhis. *British Journal of Dermatology,* 1988, **119**, 267–72.
2. Bergeron, J. R. & Stone, O. J. Koilonychia. *Archives of Dermatology,* 1967, **95**, 351.
3. Bentley-Phillips, B. & Bayles, M. A. H. Occupational koilonychia of the toe-nails. *British Journal of Dermatology,* 1971, **85**, 140.
4. Beutler, E. Tissue effects of iron deficiency. In *Iron Metabolism,* Gross, F. (ed), Springer Verlag, Berlin.
5. Crosby, D. L. & Petersen, M .J. Familial koilonychia. *Cutis,* 1989, **44** (93), 209–10.
6. Dawber, R. Occupational koilonychia. *British Journal of Dermatology,* **91,** Supplements 10, 11.
7. Dolma, T., Norboo, T., Yayha, M., Hobson, R. & Ball, K. Seasonal koilonychia in Ladakh. *Contact Dermatitis,* 1990, **22** (2), 78–80.
8. Hogan, G. R. & Jones. Koilonychia and iron deficiency in infants. *J. Paediatrics,* 1970, **77,** 1054–7.

Chapter 4
Canaliformis Deformities &
Nutritional Abnormalities

Although long, wide splits or a longitudinal hollow or canal in the nail can occur in association with malnutrition, they can occur in general or local skin diseases such as lichen planus or as a result of local trauma in the centre of the nailfold.

Malnutrition of total protein and amino acid intake, deficiency of sulphur-containing amino-acids and lack of iron have all been discussed as causes of koilonychia. As the malnutrition becomes more severe, more marked nail changes are seen. Thus, long-standing vitamin C and B2 deficiencies are also said to cause koilonychia. Various reports incriminate a negative calcium balance and deficiency of divalent ions such as magnesium with soft or even brittle and hard nails.

In children with kwashiorkor, increased nail hardness appears to be due to abnormal water increases and uneven distribution of the calcium (Robson and Brooks, 1974).

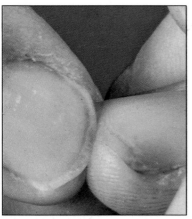 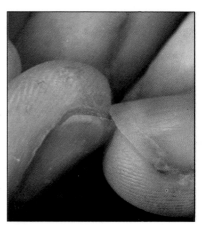

93 **94**

93 Flexibility downwards. Method of flicking the nail edge upwards and downwards. This is to measure the softness or flexibility of the free edge. Particularly useful in nutritional deficiencies.
94 Flicking nail upwards.

In the mid-1980s, quick clinical methods for studying individual trace mineral deficiencies giving rise to changes in the nails had not been clearly established, although earlier work did appear promising (Harrison & Clemena, 1972; Hopps, 1977). Sometimes, a specific abnormality may be detected in the hair or even toenails, but not the fingernails as shown for zinc (McKenzie, 1979). Under circumstances of clinical suspicion, where specific nutrient deficiency may be detected and where abnormal softness, abnormal brittleness or dystrophy is present, further clinical examination and plasma biochemistry will be necessary.

If the nail complaint is of brittleness, a standard method of springing or flicking the free nail edge, as shown, should be used. Brittle nails may occur in general systemic diseases in older patients; here there is a reduced intake of the main macro- and micro-nutrients. (*See page 64.*)

In internal medicine practice, canaliformis deformities are almost always seen in association with either changes in nutrition or local central trauma to the nail. Rare familial cases have been described. This canaliformis deformity was never found in a large group of healthy, over–75-year-old people surveyed for nutritional abnormalities by the authors.

References

1. Abdel-Aziz, A. H. & Abdel-All, H. Dystrophia unguium mediana canaliformis. *Cutis,* 1979, **23** (3), 344.
2. Harrison, W. W. & Clemena, G. G. Survey analysis of trace elements in human fingernails by spark source mass spectrometry. *Clinica Chimica Acta*, 1972, **3**, 485.
3. Heller, J. Dystrophia unguium mediana canaliformis. *Dermat. Z.*, 1928, **51**, 416.
4. Hopps, H. C. The biologic basis for using hair and nail for analyses of trace elements. *Sci. Total Environ.*, 1977, (**2**), 71.
5. Leclercq, R. Naevus striatus symetricus unguis, dystrophie mediane canaliforme de Heller ou dystrophie ungueale mediane en chevrons. *Bull. Soc. fr. Derm.,* 1964, **71**, 654.
6. McKenzie, J. M. Content of zinc in serum, urine, hair and toenails of New Zealand adults. *American Journal of Clinical Nutrition,* 1979, **32** (3), 570.
7. Robson, J. R. K. & Brooks, G. J. The distribution of calcium in finger-nails from healthy and malnourished children. *Clinica Chimca Acta,* 1974, **55**, 255.
8. Shelley, W. B. & Rawnsley, H. M. Aminogenic alopecia. *Lancet*, 1965, **ii**, 1327.
9. Sonnex, T. S., Dawber, R. P. R. & Zachary, C. B. The Nails in Pityriasis. *Rubra Pilaris: Journal of the American Academy of Dermatology,* 1986, **15**, 956–60.

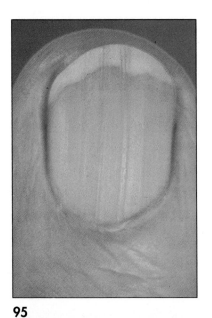

95 Nutritional deficiencies. Brittle thin nail in middle-aged woman on thyroxine replacement for surgical hypothyroidism. Note also marked longitudinal ridges and loss of lunula. Serum calcium low.

96 Early canaliformis. Very early medial canaliformis deformity in a young woman with obsessive food ideas. Little or no intake of calcium in her diet.

97 Nutritional canaliformis. Canaliformis deformity in elderly anaemic woman with combined iron, folate, mineral and protein deficiency.

98 Variation in nails. Canaliformis deformity with differences between nails.

95

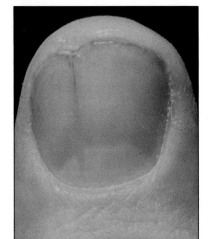

96

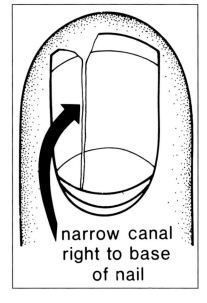

narrow canal
right to base
of nail

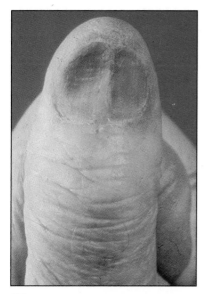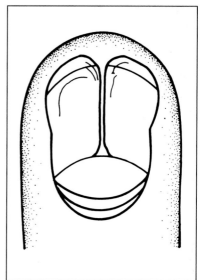

97

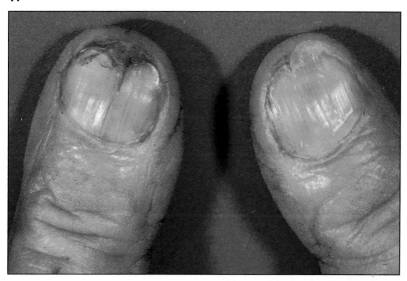

98

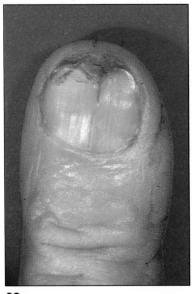

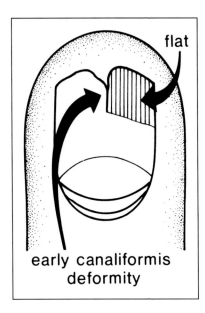

early canaliformis
deformity

99

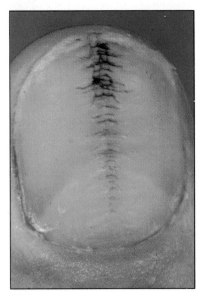

100

99 Distal deformities predominate. Dystrophic nails in a 67-year-old pensioner with nutritional deficiency secondary to extensive gastric surgery. Early canaliformis deformity of left index finger.

100 Chevron deformity. An interesting early canaliformis deformity of the pseudo-Leclercq variety. In this young clerical worker this permanent lesion is due to a very localised matrix injury some years before.

101 "Hellers" type. Hellers type of dystrophia mediana canaliformis in an elderly man with arterial disease.

102 Severe canaliformis. Dystrophia mediana canaliformis associated with abnormal discomfort in a retired elderly male living alone. Mild iron deficiency anaemia and poor nutritional state. Note oblique grooves described as chevron-shaped canaliformis deformity of Leclercq—can be traumatic as well as nutritional.

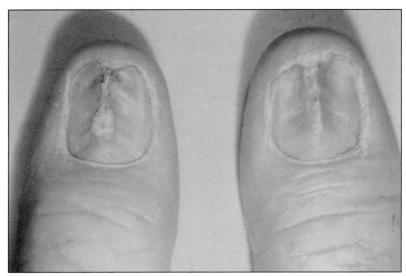

101

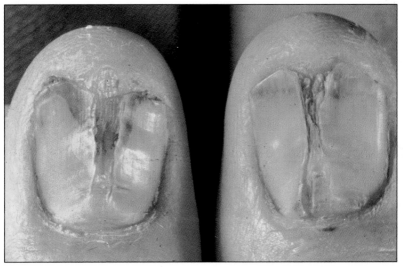

102

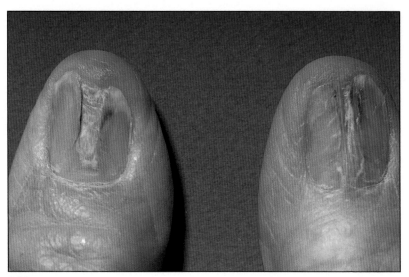

103

103 Thumbs of an elderly male living alone, who was found to have vitamin C and thiamin deficiencies, but no severe mineral problems. A classic canaliformis change opening towards base of nail.

Chapter 5
Infections Affecting Nails

Paronychias

Most of these start as the result of some form of local trauma. Although the cuticle or proximal nail fold covering the growing area of matrix cells is well adapted to resist bacterial infections, injury associated with temporary changes in immunity can allow local invasion around the nail folds.

Acute Paronychia

Acute paronychia is usually due to various forms of staphylococci. A rapid spread of inflammation with a red flare up the finger will suggest streptococcal involvement. There may be acute redness and tenderness without pus, but if the latter accumulates damage to the cells of the matrix or nail bed, the result could be some nail plate damage or dystrophy.

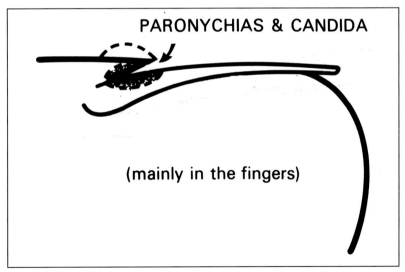

PARONYCHIAS & CANDIDA

(mainly in the fingers)

104

Chronic Paronychia

Chronic paronychia is much more common and can also be associated with more general medical disorders such as diabetes, alcoholism or autoimmune disease. In all disorders and in malignancy there is reduced immunity, as in the acute version. Low-grade redness and swelling may be present for weeks or months. This is the commonest nail complaint. Intermittent exposure to water, dirty clothes and detergents appears to be a major risk factor. Amongst women, who outnumber men by 5 to 1 in degree of exposure, the most common age of presentation is 30–60 years; apart from housewives, barmaids, nursery and laundry workers, this group seems particularly prone. Amongst males, statistics from the United Kingdom indicate that chefs, barmen, fishermen and fish-mongers are prone. There are also papers suggesting that changes in skin barrier due to allergic skin reactions in food handlers allow subsequent bacterial infection.

Various bacteria are involved, frequently including *Staphylococci* and less often *Streptococci, Coliform bacilli* and *Pseudomonas aeruginosa*. Some authors maintain that *Candida albicans* plays a crucial role in maintaining chronicity in what would otherwise be a short, sharp infection. Stone & Mullins report that chronic paronychia starts with invasion of the epidermis on the deep surface of the proximal nail fold. When chronic over several months, the paronychia, if generalised around the base of the nail, leads to various nail dystrophies. A good review of the various hypotheses relating to paronychias by Baran *et al.* stresses the complementary role of *Candida* with other bacterial infections in producing more severe and long-standing paronychias.

Recent studies have suggested that bacterial carriage in oil therapy for nails should be excluded, and damp gloves in some industrial processes may be responsible for chronic paronychias.

105   Acute bacterial infection. Acute lateral paronychia. Again in a man with brachyonychia, possibly the result of nail biting, but further examination revealed that the patient also had previously undiagnosed diabetes mellitus.
106   Acute paronychia in great toenail. Initially suggested acute tinea, but a bead of pus grew staphylococcus.
107   Herpetic whitlow. Frequently seen in nursing staff. When severe, gives onycholysis or nail shedding (La Rossa & Hamilton, 1971).

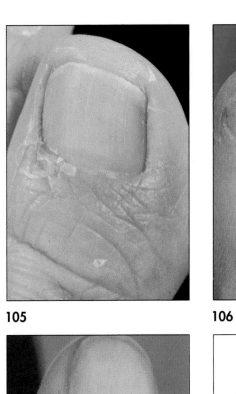

105

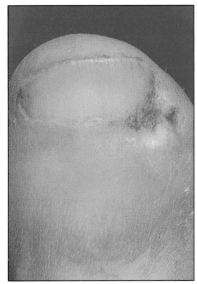

106

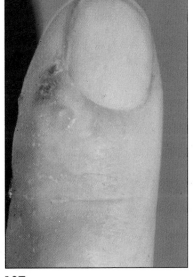

107

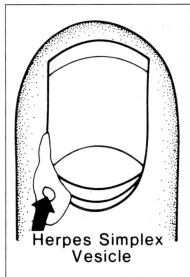

Herpes Simplex
Vesicle

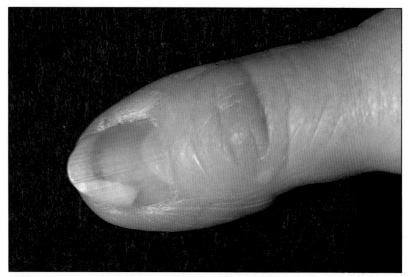

108

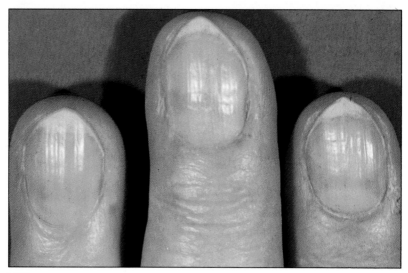

109

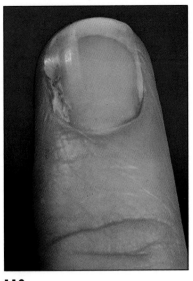
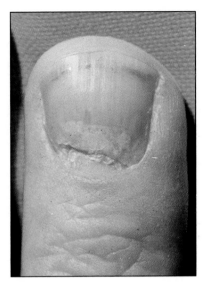

110   **111**

108   End result of previous lateral paronychia.

109   Mild healing paronychia. Healing paronychia in 23-year-old female clerical worker. Note old lesion on right side of finger.

110   Chronicity in one finger. Chronic and persistent low-grade paronychia in a woman trainee air-force chef. Note care and attention to rest of manicure.

111   Healing with dystrophy. Healed paronychia in 36-year-old married woman with six children. Consequent nail dystrophy—when grown further could be described as onychomadesis (division across nail).

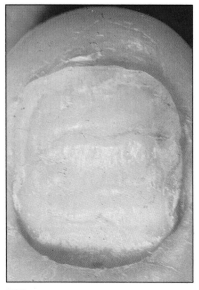

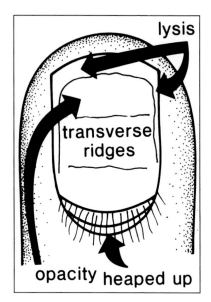

112

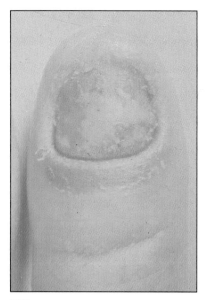

113

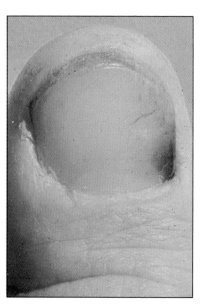

114

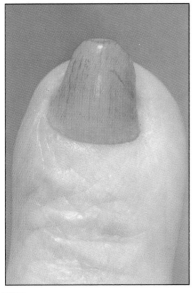
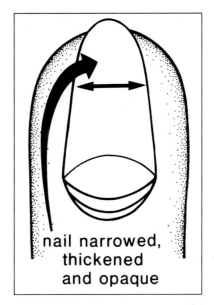

nail narrowed,
thickened
and opaque

115

112 Chronic paronychia—marked nail ridging. Mixed infections. Note nail dystrophy and lysis on all edges. Transverse ridges on nail.

113 Repeated infections. Acute bacterial infections are common in housewives with hands frequently immersed in water, or where general immunity is impaired.

114 Small lateral lesion with pigment. Lateralised local small area of chronic paronychia leading to nail changes distally.

115 Distortion of nails. Chronic paronychia with chronic nail dystrophy in a 42-year-old housewife on long-term corticosteroid medication for asthma.

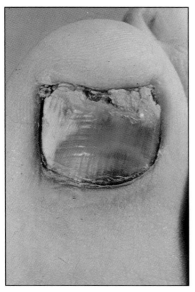

116 Chronic *Pseudomonas.* Chronic infection in great toenail bed— *Pseudomonas* infection giving characteristic green colour; probably a complication of previous subungual haematoma.

116

References

1. Baran, R., Barth, J. & Dawber, R. Nail disorders: Differential diagnosis and signs & treatment. 1991, Martin Dunitz, Gillingham, Kent.
2. Editorial: Chronic Paronychias. *British Medical Journal II,* 1975, 460.
3. Leyden, J. J., McGinley, K. J., Kates, S. G. & Myung, K. B. Subungual bacteria of the hand. *Infect. Control Hosp. Epidemiol.*, 1975, **10,** 451–4.
4. Pottinger, J., Burns, S. & Manske, C. Bacterial carriage by artificial versus natural nails. *Am. J. Infect. Control.* 1989, **17** (16), 340–4.

Fungal Infections & Onychomycoses

In 1990, a survey for fungal infections was carried out involving 9000 adults in the United Kingdom. A questionnaire and photographs were used to identify nail dystrophies.

The results of the survey revealed a prevalence of dermatophyte nail infection of 2.8% in men and 2.6% in women. In the group aged 16–34 years, the prevalence rate was 1.3%; this increased to 2.4% in the group aged 35–50 years, and to 4.7% in those aged 55 years or over.

Of those found to have onychomycosis, 27% had sought advice from a chiropodist, and less than 12% had consulted a specialist. These results suggested that nearly 1.2 million people in the UK had a fungal nail infection, and the majority had not sought medical advice, although over 80% stated that they would do so if they were aware that their nail disorder was of fungal origin.

These fungal elements, which affect the fingernails less commonly, are likely to be *Candida albicans*, but 70% of the damage in the toenails results from dermatophytes. The earliest sign of fungus of the fingernail will usually be small, asymmetrical, white patches or lifting of one edge of the nail plate. Subsequently, the mycosis may spread to involve the whole nail plate with slowly increasing opacity, thickening and distortion. As the integrity of the nail is damaged, both air and dirt may enter the split layers of the nail

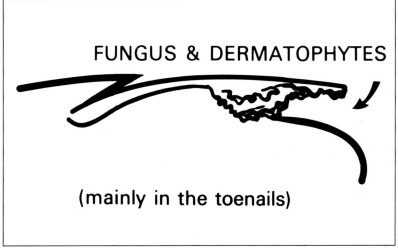

FUNGUS & DERMATOPHYTES

(mainly in the toenails)

117

plate to give a variety of appearances. These include white nails, brown nails and thickened and black nails. Gradual lifting of the nail plate occurs with lateral or distal onycholysis. In more severe infections with a heavy burden of fungus, the whole nail may be shed. If the clinical appearance is not characteristic, clippings or scrapings of the nail should be taken to establish the diagnosis.

In most developing and tropical countries, where bare-footedness is common, minor nail infections are endemic and the types of fungi usually related to those prevalent in that geographic area. Lists of common dermatophytes are included in the toenails section of this book (Chapter 15).

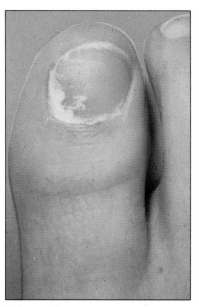

118

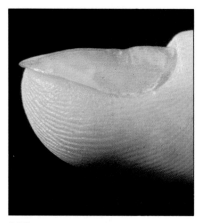

119

118 "Tinea". Onychomycosis at base of great toenail.
119 Chronic *Trichophyton*. Lateral view of chronic *Trichophyton* infection in the index finger of young housewife with two small babies.
120 Yellow great toenail scopulariopsis. Tinea of toenail. Scopulariopsis brevicaulis. Note that the second toe is affected.
121 Chronic fungus finger. Tinea of the fingernail of a hotel washing-up maid.

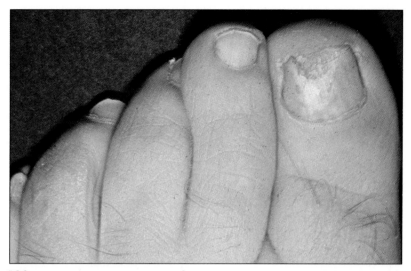

120

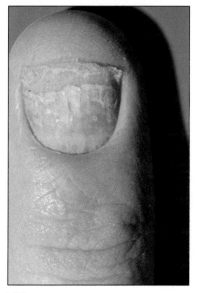

121

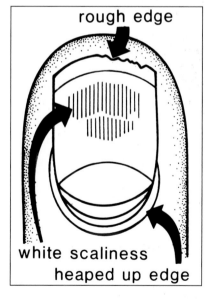

rough edge

white scaliness
heaped up edge

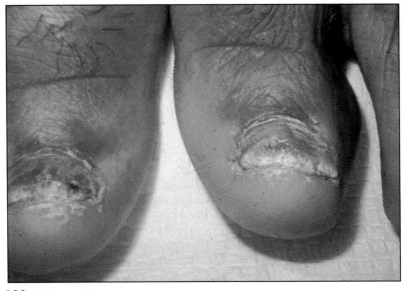

122

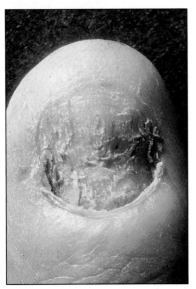

123

122 Chronic toenail infection. Tinea pedis. Note dystrophy mainly at distal or leading edge.

123 End-stage dystrophy. Severe end-stage nail secondary to *Trichophyton rubum.*

124 Reduced immunity. Elderly male with chronic candidiasis now under control but leading to severe nail dystrophy. Always suspect diabetes mellitus and endocrine diseases.

125 Continuing infection. Long-term chronic fungal infection (*Trichophyton*) in toenail leading to general nail dystrophy.

126 Proximal nail not infected. Dermatophytic onychomycosis. Note that the disorder starts at leading edge and works back up the nail.

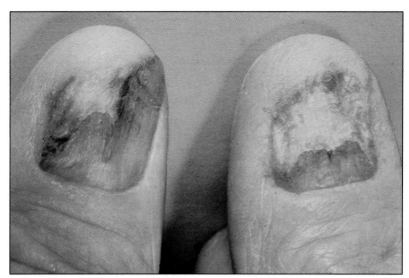

124

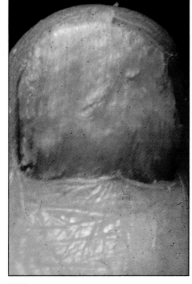

125

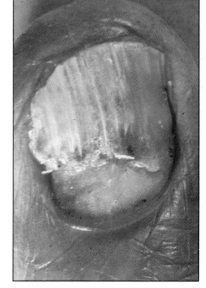

126

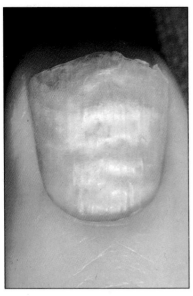

127

127 *Leukonychia onychomycosis.* More severe form of fungal infection in nail. Long-standing disease leads to complete opacity.

128 Nail marker of endocrinopathy. Chronic candidiasis affecting 19-year-old male with autoimmune endocrinopathy (including adrenal and thyroid deficiencies).

129 Familial nail involvement. Very severe *Candida* infection in one of two brothers with autoimmune endocrine disease (adrenals and thyroid failure)—severe *Candida* infections may be an important marker of endocrine hypofunction.

130 Hypertrophy secondary to chronic *Candida.*

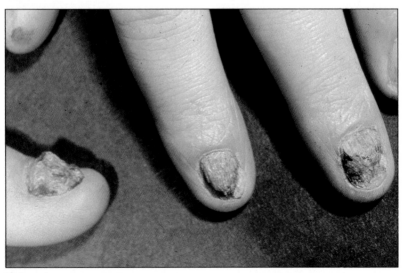

128

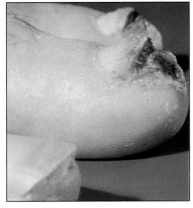 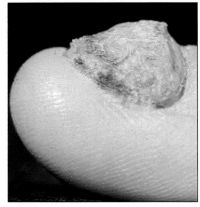

129 **130**

References

1. Davies, R. R., Everall, J. D. & Hamilton, E. Mycological and clinical evaluation of griseofulvin for chronic onychomycosis. *British Medical Journal,* 1967, **2,** 464.

2. Moore, M. K. The infection of human skin and nail by *Scytalidium* Species. *Current topics in Medical Mycology,* 1992, **4,** 1-42.

3. Monod, M., Baudraz-Rosselet, F., Ramelet, A. A. & Frenk, E. Direct mycological examination in dermatology: a comparison of different methods. *Dermatologica,* 1989, **179** (4), 183–6.

4. Nicholls, D. S. & Midglet, G. Onychomycosis caused by Trichophyton equinum. *Clin. Exp. Dermatol.,* 1989, **14** (96), 464–5.

5. Patki, A. H. & Mehta, J. M. Pterygium unguis in a patient with recurrent type 2 lepra reaction. *Cutis,* 1989, **44** (4), 311–2.

6. Ramesh, V., Reddy, B. S. & Singh, R. Onychomycosis. *International Journal of Dermatology,* 1983, **22** (3) 148.

7. Roberts, D. T. Prevalence of dermatophyte. Onychomycosis in the United Kingdom. *British Journal of Dermatology,* 1992, **126,** Suppl 39, 23–7.

8. Todd, P., Garioch, J., Rademaker, M., Susskind, W., Gemett, C. & Thomson, J. Pachyonychia congenita complicated by hidradenitis suppurativa: a family study. *British Journal of Dermatology,* 1990, **123** (5), 663–6.

9. Tosti, A., Guerra, L., Morelli, R., Bardazzi, F. & Fanti, P. A. Role of foods in the pathogenesis of chronic paronychia. *Journal of the American Academy of Dermatology,* 1992, **27** (5, Pt 1), 706–10.

10. Walshe, M. M. & English, M. P. Fungous diseases of Britain. *British Journal of Dermatol,* 1966, **78,** 198.

HIV Infections of Nails

There are no specifically identifiable signs or appearances in the nails of people with Human Immunodeficiency Virus (HIV). As the deficiency is a generalised one, a wide variety of appearances is possible. Surprisingly, not all nails are affected or involved.

The following appear to be the most commonly reported nail signs presenting in persons infected with HIV:

- Proximal white subungual onychomycosis.
- Superficial white onychomycosis on several nails.
- A destructive, almost gramulomatous-like appearance, similar to moderately severe psoriasis, which it mimics.
- Melanotic or pigmented streaks and longitudinal lines.

Candida albicans and *Trichophytons*—particularly *T. rubrum*—are the organisms most commonly found in the nails of HIV-positive patients. Occasionally, other pigmented patches on the hands or feet are associated with pigmented streaks or bands in the nails. Squamous cell and other secondary malignancies have also been reported in the nail beds of HIV-positive patients.

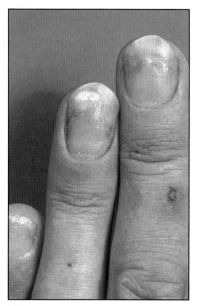

131 & 132 A young man in his 20s, not previoulsy known to be HIV-positive, was admitted with pulmonary lesions. Note poor immune state and infected lesion on finger.
133 & 134 HIV-positive male in his 30s presenting with changes in nails. Middle and ring fingernails shown.

131

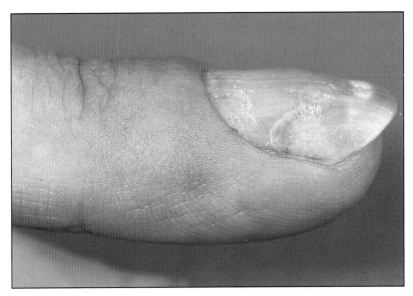

132

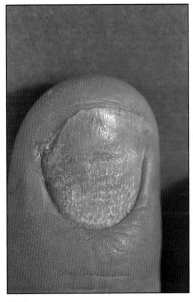

133

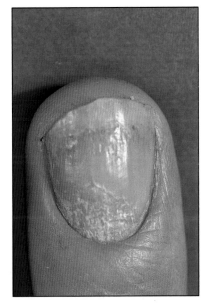

134

References

1. Chandrasekar, P. H. Nail discoloration and human immunodeficiency virus infection. *Am. J. Med.,* April 1989, **86** (4), 506–7.
2. Dompmartin, D., Dompmartin, A., Deluol, A. M., Grosshans, E. & Couland, J. P. Onychomycosis and AIDS. Clinical and laboratory findings in 62 patients. *International Journal of Dermatology,* 1990, **29** (5), 337–9.
3. Daniel, C. R. 3d, Norton, L. A. & Scher, R. K. The spectrum of nail disease in patients with human immunideficiency virus infection. *Journal of the American Academy of Dermatology,* 1992, **27** (1), 93–7.
4. Gallais, V., Lacour, J. P., Perrin, C., Ghanem, G., Bodokh, I. & Ortonne, J. P. Acral hyperpigmented macules and longitudinal melanonychia in AIDS patients. *British Journal of Dermatology,* 1992, **126** (4), 387–91.
5. Prose, N. S., Abson, K. G. & Scher, R. K. Disorders of the nails and hair associated with human immunodeficiency virus infection. *International Journal of Dermatology,* 1992, **31** (7), 453–7.

Chapter 6
Altered Circulation

Increasingly, disorders of more affluent, westernised societies—such as hypertension, diabetes mellitus, obesity and hypercholesterolaemia with consequent atheroma—are spreading to all parts of the world. Turbulence and gravitational forces lead to increasing atheroma of the aortic arch and bifarcation of the aorta and leg vessels. With greater longevity, impaired blood supply to the toes may show as nail dystrophies or opacities secondary to mycoses. Pigment on the fingernails from nicotine smoking is seen with rough whitened toenails and skin ischaemia. In contrast to the male preponderance for toenail signs of leg ischaemia, women more commonly present with nail changes in the hands.

Changes in the nails with thinning and brittleness or a ground-glass opacity may occur secondary to atheroma. In every such patient seen by one of the authors, general physical examination revealed other evidence of atheroma. Signs of leg ischaemia, electrocardiographic changes, bruits over various arteries and "kinked-carotid" arteries were always present. The only exception to this appears in cases where arm arterial emboli break up and are not removed surgically. Under these circumstances, one sees localised and chronic changes in digital blood flow secondary to narrowing in the ulnar artery or palmar arch. Such patients are seen rarely even in a busy teaching hospital.

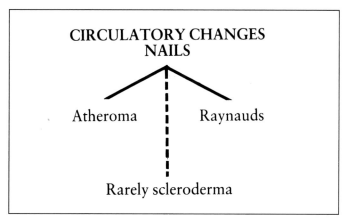

135

Traumatic injury to the toenails, common in industrial workers in the tropics and leisure activitists in temperature zones, and taking more than 8 months to grow out along the nail, suggests atheroma further "upstream".

Raynaud's disease or episodic vascular spasm precipitated by cold may come on slowly over many years—or often develop slowly from puberty. It may affect digital arteries, with little or no skin disease associated with the early nail changes. As it may be symptomatic for developing autoimmune disease, relevant tests are necessary and a careful history essential.

References

1. Edwards, E. A. Nail changes in functional and organic arterial disease. *New England Journal of Medicine*, 1948, **239**, 362.
2. Mahler, F., Saner, H., Wurbel, H. & Flammer, J. Local cooling test for clinical capillaroscopy in Raynaud's phenomenon, unstable angina, and vasospastic visual disorders. *Vasa,* 1989, **18** (3), 201–4.
3. Samman, P. D. & Strickland, B. Abnormalities of the finger nails associated with impaired peripheral blood supply. *British Journal of Dermatology,* 1962, **74**, 163.
4. Strickland, B. & Urquhart, W. Digital arteriography, with reference to nail dystrophy. *British Journal of Radiology,* 1963, **36**, 465.

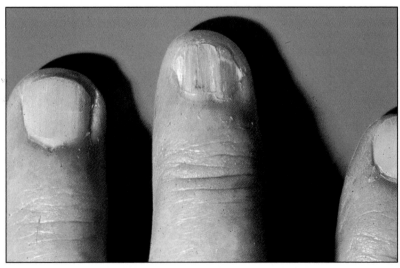

136

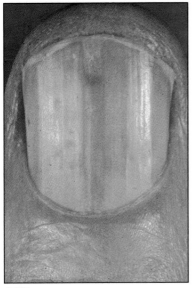
137

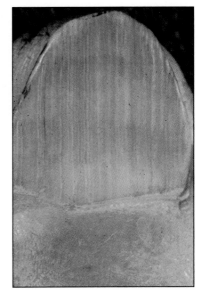
138

136 Digital artery only. Nail dystrophy secondary to injury to right digital artery of the middle finger of a young male.

137 Generalised atheroma. Left thumbnail from a 69-year-old diabetic man who has severe generalised atheroma. Bilateral sympathectomy to feet; left hand often cold. Note small central onycholysis in leading edge—reddening of the centre of the nail, extending through the lunula and the small, abnormal pits to the left of the mid-line. No evidence of psoriasis.

138 Severe arch atheroma. Gross aortic arch atheroma with dystrophic, flattened and opaque nail.

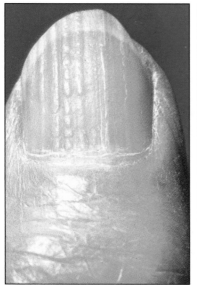
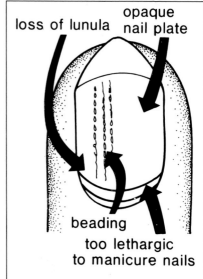

loss of lunula

opaque nail plate

beading

too lethargic to manicure nails

139

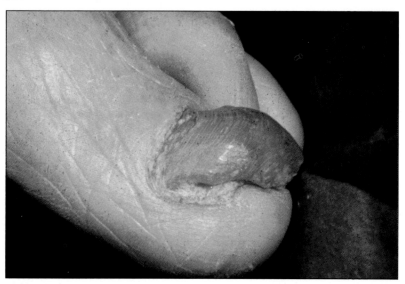

140

IMPAIRED CIRCULATION IN NAILS

(1) **Atheroma — opacity — gradual loss**
(2) **Raynaud's — brittle — loss — onycholysis pterygia — long ridges**
(3) **Scleroderma — + soft tissues**
(4) **Yellow nail syndrome — lymphatic abnormalities**

141

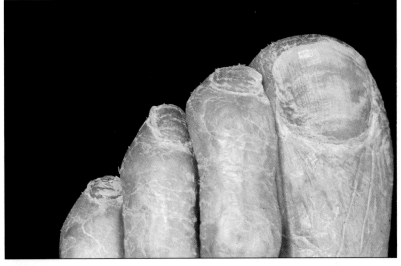

142

139 Generalised atheroma. Thumbnail of a 76-year-old woman in failing health secondary to coronary artery disease and chronic left ventricular failure. Note slight cyanosis, opacity of nail, marked beading and loss of lunula.

140 Leg ischaemia. Arterial insufficiency disguised by onychogryphosis. Note ischaemic changes in skin of great toe.

141 Impaired circulation.

142 Ischaemia foot. A 65-year-old man with ischaemic skin changes typical of severe reduction in blood supply. Note also scaling from dry beri-beri with abnormal TPP level.

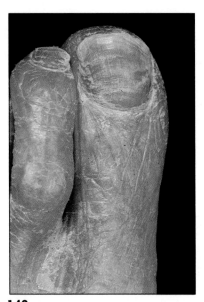

143

143   Toenail ischaemia. Same 65-year-old man with absent foot pulses. Gross ischaemic changes in great toe.

144   Raynaud's nails.

145   Onycholysis in a woman with severe Raynaud's disorder.

146   Atheromatous changes affecting nails and skin in middle-aged Maori male labourer with diabetes mellitus.

147   Early scleroderma. Nail in early scleroderma. The only changes are some "pointing" in terminal pulp and opacity of nail.

148   Lifelong Raynaud's. Severe Raynaud's disease with loss of toenails.

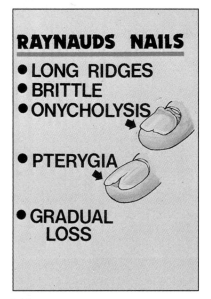

RAYNAUDS NAILS

- LONG RIDGES
- BRITTLE
- ONYCHOLYSIS
- PTERYGIA
- GRADUAL LOSS

144

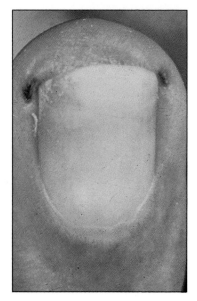

145

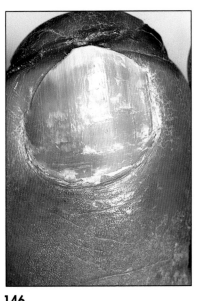

146

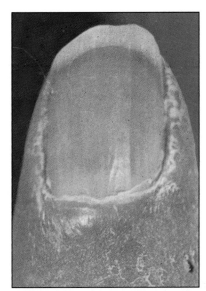

147

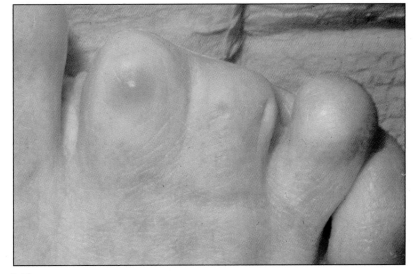

148

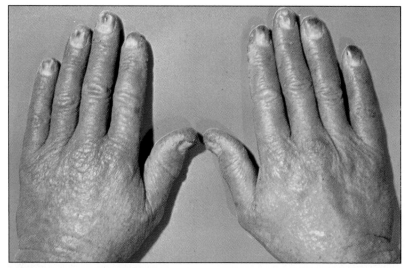

149

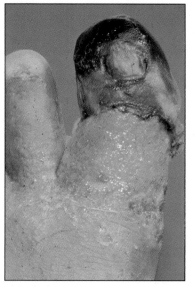

150

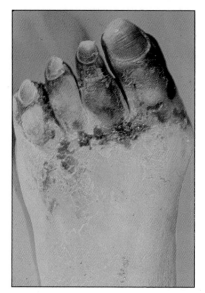

151

96

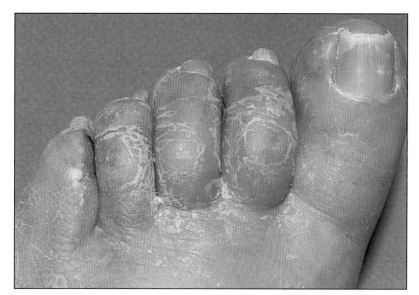

152

149 Scleroderma. Some nails show pigment. Hand colour very dusky and pigmented due to secondary circulation impairment.

150 Temporary nail damage. Early frostbite—only nail of great toe will be lost. As matrix cells are damaged, permanent nail dystrophy remains.

151 More marked frostbite with damage to matrix cells and toenail beds of all digits.

152 Moderate frostbite of foot on older man. 3rd & 4th toenails will later show damage. (2nd & 5th nails already mycotic.)

153 Autoimmune disease. Digital artery thrombosis in an old lady with rheumatoid arthritis and positive LE cells, leading to gangrene of fingertip and loss of nail.

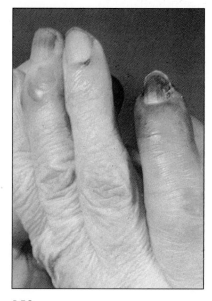

153

Chapter 7
Nail Trauma

Minor Injuries

Single, smaller injuries to the nail plate may result in fracture of the capillaries supplying the matrix cells. The most minor may later show as a tiny white spot, which in turn grows outward over subsequent months.

More severe injuries, with localised connections of blood giving rise to a visible haematoma, may cause growth arrest lines or, if severe, avulsion and loss of nail. It is customary practice to release the blood by a small "burr hole", perhaps reducing pressure on matrix cells.

The management of crush injuries to the nail alone or of the fingers calls for specialised skill, preferably in a hand unit, and is well discussed by Michon & Delagoutte (1980) and by Iselin (1980).

Occupational Injuries

Repeated injury from either chemical or mechanical trauma can be identified from the history or from the particular unskilled labouring work involved. Mechanically driven tools, "Flymo" power lawnmowers or "Weedeaters" worked close to bare feet can inflict permanent nail injury.

Other Nail Trauma

Nail-biting in adults is usually a failure to resolve personality conflicts and a lack of feeling of self-worth late in life. Habit tics of various types will damage one single nail only. Excessive anxiety or various habit traits may lead to repeated pushing back of the cuticle with manicure equipment, "orange sticks" or even the teeth. Such repetitive minor trauma can lead to transverse lines, nail opacities or splitting of the free edge of the nail.

"Hang nails" are torn or narrow strips of the horny epidermis, split up from the lateral nail fold. Failure to care for the cuticle, nail-biting or using the teeth to push back the quick may lead to an increased frequency of damage.

154   White spot of slight trauma 3 months previously. No nail dystrophy.
155   Thumb injured in bicycle accident in childhood. Now shows brachonychia, "senile" longitudinal striations in middle life.
156   Blow to finger and changes from mid-nail bed injury several weeks later.

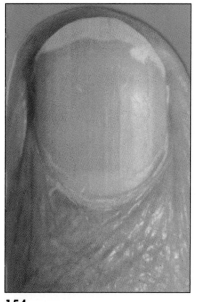

154

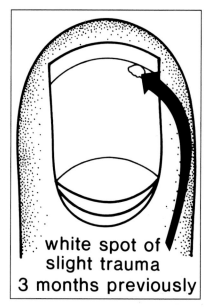

white spot of slight trauma 3 months previously

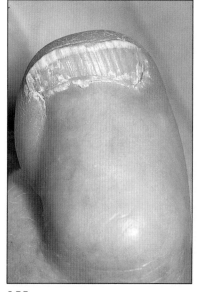

155

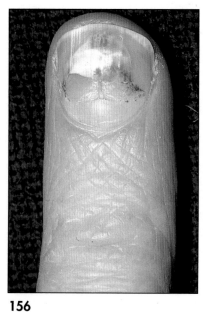

156

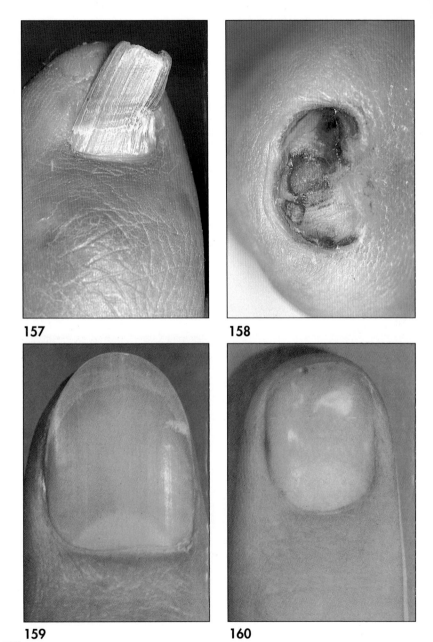

157

158

159

160

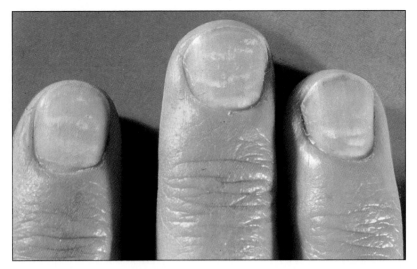

161

157 "Industrial" accident to proximal nail bed 3 months previously in a Maori seaman.

158 Hallux nail bed trauma whilst working barefoot—traumatic lysis of nail.

159 Mild unremembered injury. Normal nail with small old (white) injury spot on left border. Female scientist in her 20s.

160 Frequent knocking of hands. Mild trauma resulting in one large and several small white patches.

161 Occupational injury. Multiple small injuries over 3 or 4 months in a young woman working at basket-making. Many small white spots, whereas only a few are seen in "normal" nails.

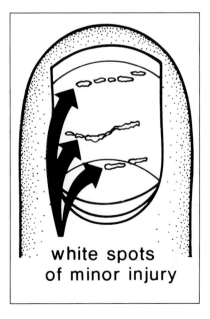

white spots of minor injury

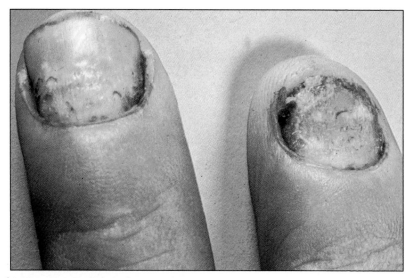

162

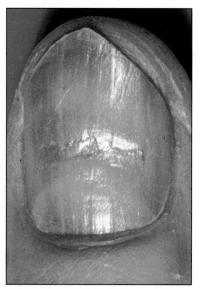

162 Occupational trauma. Dystrophy and minor repeated chemical injury to eponychium or nail fold in a factory worker in the car battery trade.

163 Car door injury. Fingernail of a senior nursing sister whose finger was lightly jammed in a car door. Partially disguised by nail varnish; can be a growth arrest line.

163

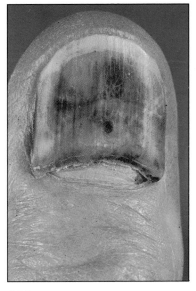

164

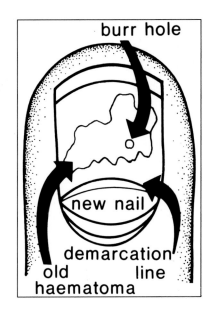

164 Subungual haematoma. Thumb-nail of middle-aged male who sustained moderate trauma from a hammer injury some weeks previously. Note hole drilled in attempt to release the haematoma.

165 Healing subungual haematoma. Healing phase of thumbnail in photograph 164 taken 8 weeks later, showing somewhat increased rate of growth of new nail plate.

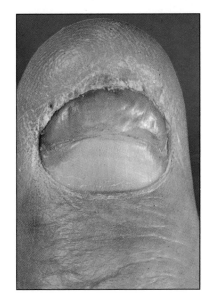

165

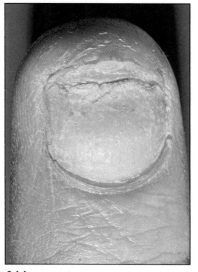

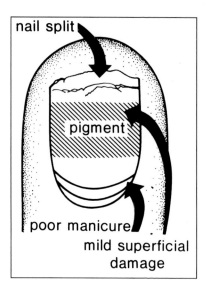

166

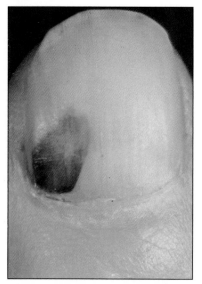

167

166 Major occupational trauma. Nail dystrophy due to repeated work trauma in printing trade.

167 Repeated nail bleeding. Mild trauma leading to subungual haematoma in a patient with long-standing diabetes. Positive Hess or cuff test on arm and normal platelets suggests capillary fragility.

168 Childhood trauma. Trauma to middle fingertip, including nail matrix, from an injury in early childhood.

169 Dorsal view. Moderate trauma to nail some years previously. Pigment probably due to low-grade inflammatory bowel disease.

170 Lateral view of old injury. Moderate trauma to nail some years previously. Pigment probably due to low-grade inflammatory bowel disease.

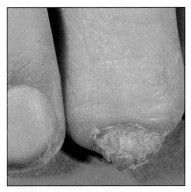

168

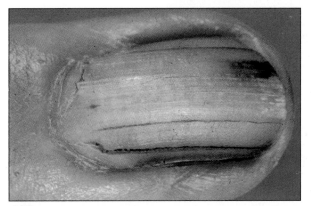

169

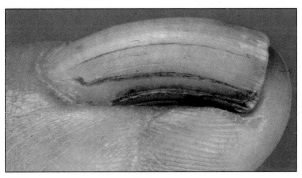

170

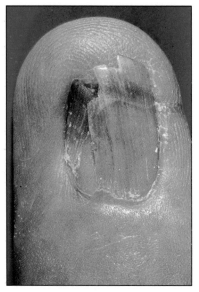 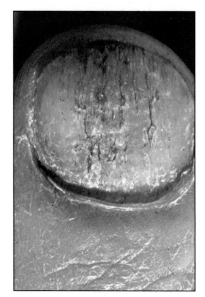

171   **172**

171 Fingertip trauma. Small left-sided pterygium in the fingernail of a labouring man who had suffered a stroke from severe arterial disease.

172 Repetitive trauma. Nail dystrophy due to repetitive work trauma experienced by wire worker.

173 Recent cutting injury illustrating the dangers of not using foot protection when using a circular cutting "Flymo" lawn-mower.

174 Complete recent avulsion hallux toenail.

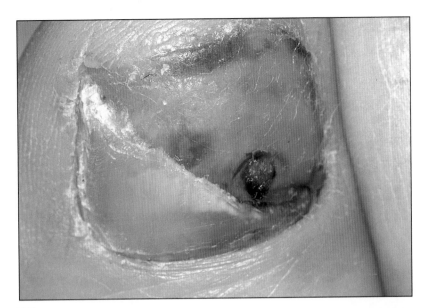

173

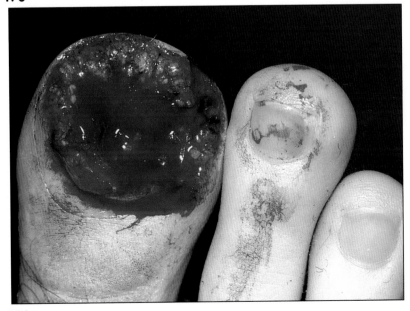

174

References

1. Chudnofsky, C. R. & Sebastian, S. Special wounds. Nail bed, plantar puncture, and cartilage. *Emergency Medicine Clinics of North America,* **10** (4), 801–22.
2. Farrington, G. H. Subungual haematoma—An evaluation of treatment. *British Medical Journal,* 1964, **1**, 742.
3. Guy, R. J. The etiologies and mechanisms of nail bed injuries. *Hand. Clin.,* 1990, **6** (1), 9–19.
4. Johnson, R. K. Nailplasty. *Plastic and Reconstructive Surgery,* 1971, **47**, 275.
5. Michon, J. & Delagoutte, J. P. (p. 81) & Iselin, M. (p. 83). In *The Nail,* Pierre, M. (ed). Churchill Livingstone, London, 1981.
6. Samman, P. D. A traumatic nail dystrophy produced by a habit tic. *Archives of Dermatology,* 1963, **88**, 895.
7. Samman, P. D. Nail disorders caused by external influences. *Journal of the Society of Cosmetic Chemistry,* 177, **8**, 351.
8. Stone, O. J. & Mullins, J. F. The distal course of nail matrix haemorrhage *Archives of Dermatology,* 1963, **88**,186.

Chapter 8
Other Onychodystrophies

Lifting of the nail plate off the underlying nailbed is literally a lysis of the nail, hence the term "onycholysis". Minor degrees are commonly seen in response to drug-induced photosensitivity and occupational causes, including local trauma, but for the primary care health worker or practitioner, thyrotoxicosis or other dermatological disorders such as psoriasis or lichen planus declare themselves by the associated skin lesions. Rare congenital onycholysis may persist into adult life, as may also happen in disorders such as lichen striatus, but here other nail dystrophies in the other fingernails are usual.

In the uncommon but striking "yellow nail" syndrome, and in unusual general conditions such as Stevens–Johnson and Lyells syndromes, cytotoxic treatment and some cases of cardiac arrest, more severe separation of the nail is called onychomadesis.

Shedding and dystrophies are common in the affected nail in paronychia, especially if chronic or troublesome, and of course in generalised skin diseases such as psoriasis, bullous disease and lichen planus.

In a review of 113 cases of idiopathic onycholysis of the great toenail, Baran & Badillet (1982) found trauma to be a major aetiological factor. In many of their cases, trauma was found to be associated with the wearing of inappropriate shoes.

Other nail dystrophies (due to chemical injury), such as tetracycline reactions, pityriasis rubra pilaris and lammellar splitting (onychoschizia) of the nails, are less commonly seen than rough thickening of the nail plate. Known by skin specialists as trachyonychia (rough nails), the broken roughened surface is usually caused by chemical injury, some industrial dermatoses or, rarely, lichen planus. In the majority of these nail dystrophies, note should be taken of the following:

• A careful occupational and social history.
• Associated skin conditions, which will usually help with the diagnosis.

Nail dystrophies are said to occur in malnutrition, but when associated with pellagra, beri-beri, scurvy or multiple micronutrient deficiency states it is our experience that the nails are usually thin and brittle.

Classified below are a variety of nail plate changes, including:

• Onycholysis—lysis or lifting of nail.
• Onychomadesis—shedding of distal part after severe growth arrest.
• Pterygia of nails—often due to lichen planus or nail trauma.

Relatively common causes of nail lysis or lifting are set out in Table 2 (overleaf).

In the toenails, minor trauma is always a major factor, and can be the result of forced walking in inappropriate footwear. A study of the shoes can be rewarding.

In other skin diseases associated with onycholysis, the cause of the nail lifting and shedding is usually obvious as is seen in contact dermatitis and chemical and solvent injuries.

TABLE 2. *Commonly seen causes of onychodystrophies leading to lysis of nails*

Common causes of onycholysis:

- Trauma
- Thyrotoxicosis
- Psoriasis
- Long nails and trauma

Cutaneous (less common):

- Dermatitis (often contact)
- Congenital nail syndromes
- Drug eruptions (Bleomycin, Doxorubicin)
  —and other oncology treatments.
- Side effects of treatment and photosensitivity
  to drugs (Tetracyclines, Chlorpromazine)

Local and chemical causes:

- Occupational
- Chemical: alkalis, solvents, cosmetics

175 Onycholysis from anaemia. Distal onycholysis in 59-year-old woman with breast cancer and recent anaemia from secondary bone marrow involvement. Nutrition and serum albumen normal. Note: there is no koilonychia.

176 Lateral onycholysis. Three months' history of lateral onycholysis in young male dentist. Possibly a result of hand trauma.

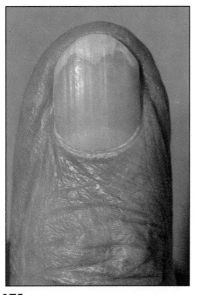
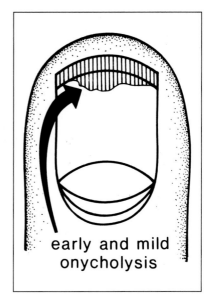

early and mild
onycholysis

175

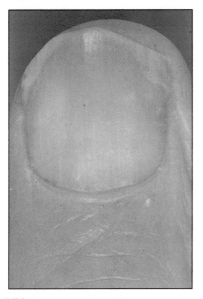

early lateral
onycholysis

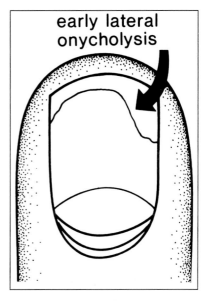

176

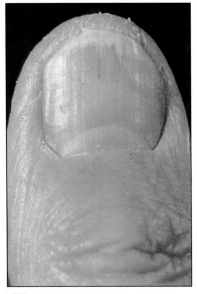

177

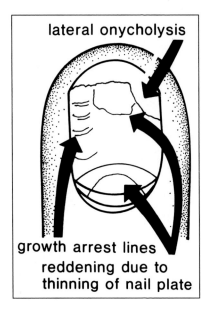

lateral onycholysis

growth arrest lines
reddening due to
thinning of nail plate

177 Multiple changes. Nail changes with lateral onycholysis, thinning of nail plate and growth arrest lines in a 72-year-old diabetic with a long-standing requirement for insulin. The only general medical abnormalities found were indifferently controlled diabetes mellitus and very poorly fitting upper and lower dentures.

178 Onycholysis of unknown cause. Unusual onycholysis with no other abnormality other than long-standing diabetes.

179 Multiple changes. "Beading" on fingernail of hypothyroid male on treatment with thyroxine. Note lack of beading near lunula and failure of care, suggesting lapse in treatment.

180 Psoriatic onycholysis. More severe onycholysis due to psoriasis in a 34-year-old male technician. Only other skin lesions were pitting in other nails and lesions in scalp hair.

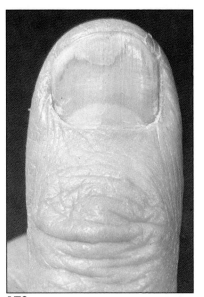

178

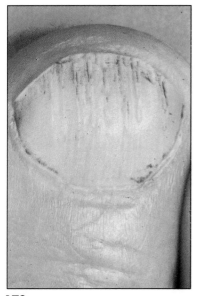

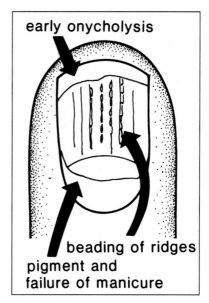

early onycholysis

beading of ridges
pigment and
failure of manicure

179

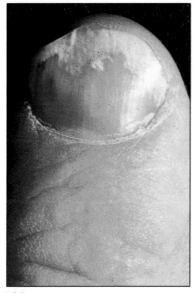

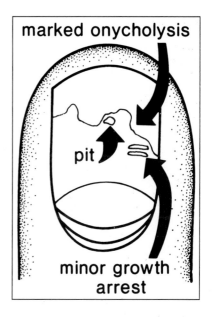

marked onycholysis

pit

minor growth
arrest

180

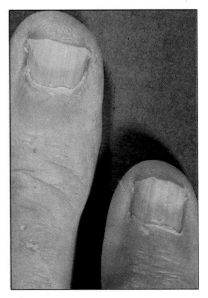
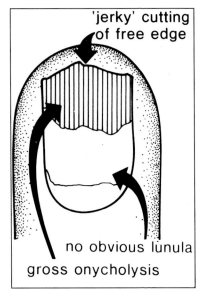

'jerky' cutting of free edge

no obvious lunula

gross onycholysis

181

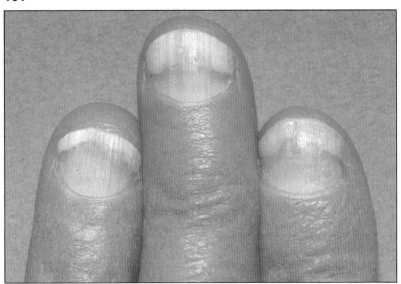

182

181 Thyrotoxic onycholysis. Untreated thyrotoxicosis in a young middle-aged woman with 1 year of increasing symptoms. No evidence of psoriasis. Note "jerky" cutting of free edge.

182 Terminal lysis from reaction to combined tetracylines and tricylic antidepressive drugs.

183 Half-and-half onycholysis. Unexplained lysis of most nails of a middle-aged woman. No evidence of psoriasis, but needs follow-up.

184 Widespread non-psoriatic onycholysis in a woman in her 60s— drug-induced by tetracylines and chlorpromazine.

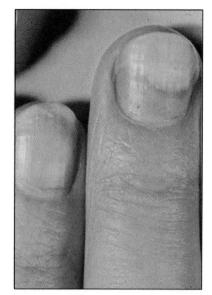

183

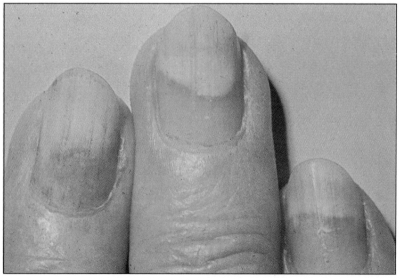

184

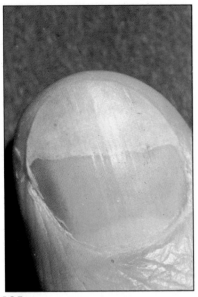

185 Severe thyrotoxic onycholysis. Half-and-half onycholysis seen in a middle-aged woman with severe thyrotoxicosis.

186 Unknown dystrophy. Unknown terminal nail dystrophy—no known psoriasis or other skin condition. This must be watched in the next few years.

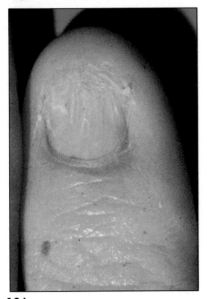

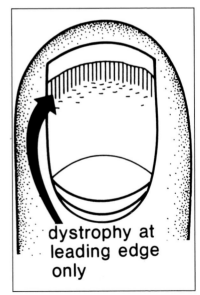

dystrophy at leading edge only

187 Ventral spur. Central ventral spur on underside of nail only—not associated with any known disease. This is a very exceptional condition.

188 Nail dystrophy. Microcryptosis in smallest toenail.

189 Lichen planus. Distal nail dystrophy in young female with lichen planus.

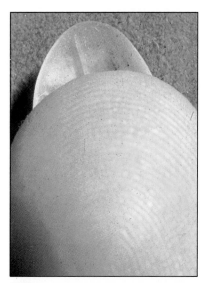

187

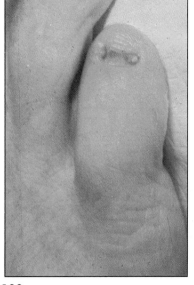

188

189

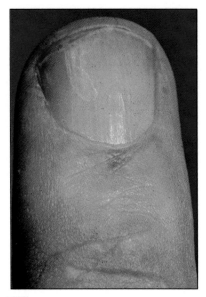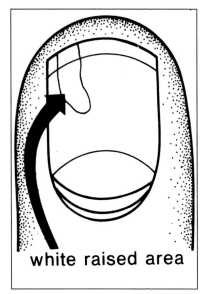

white raised area

190

190   Early lichen planus. Very early lichen planus, giving rise to odd, raised, white distal area.

References

1. Baran, R. & Badillet, G. Primary onycholysis of toenails (113 cases). *British Journal of Dermatology,* 1982, **106** (5), 529.
2. Bjellerup, M. Nail changes induced by penicillamine. *Acta Derm. Venereol.* (Stockholm), 1989, **69** (4), 339–41.
3. Dawber, R. P. R., Samman, P. D. & Bottoms, E. Finger nail growth in idiopathic and psoriatic onycholysis. *British Journal of Dermatology,* 1971, **85**, 558.
4. Eastwood, J. B., Curtis, J. R., Smith, E. K. M. & Wardener, H. E. de. Shedding of nails apparently induced by the administration of large amount of cephaloridine and cloxacillin in two anephoric patients. *British Journal of Dermatology,* 1969, **81,** 750.

5. Frank, S. B., Coher, H. J. & Minkin, W. Photo-onycholysis due to tetracycline hydrochloride and doxycycline. *Archives of Dermatology,* 1971, **103,** 520.
6. Garioch, J. & Simpson, N. B. Etretinate and severe nail plate dystrophies. *Clin. Exp. Dermatol.*, 1989, **14** (3), 261–2.
7. McCormack, L. S., Elgart, M. L. & Turner, M. L. Benoxaprofen-induced photo-onycholysis. *Journal of the American Academy of Dermatology,* 1982, **7** (5), 678.
8. Myers, M., Storino, W. & Barsky, S. Lichen striatus with nail dystrophy. *Archives of Dermatology,* 1978, **114** (6), 964.
9. Ray, I. Onycholysis. *Archives of Dermatology,* 1963, **88,** 181.
10. Sowden, J. M. Cartwright, P. H., Green, J. R. & Leonard, J. N. Isolated lichen planus of the nails associated with primary biliary cirrhosis. *British Journal of Dermatology,* 1989, **121** (5), 659–62.
11. Swan, R. H. Oral lichen planis with associated nail changes. *Journal of Oral Medicine,* 1982, **37** (1), 23.
12. Tan, S. V., Berth-Jones, J. & Burns, D. A. Lichen planus and photo-onycholysis induced by quinine. *Clin. Exp. Dermatol.,* 1989, **14** (4), 335.
13. Torras, H., Manuel Mascaro J. Jr., Mascaro, J. M. Photo-onycholysis caused by clorazepate dipotassium. *Journal of the American Academy of Dermatology,* 1989, **21** (96), 1304–5.
14. Wilson, J. W. Paronychia and onycholysis. Aetiology and therapy. *Archives of Dermatology,* 1965, **92,** 726.

Chapter 9
Psoriasis

Minimal nail changes

Changes in the nails, if untreated, are slowly progressive. They may first show themselves by tiny punctate depressions called pits.

Minimal changes are a few tiny pitted holes or some lysis at the edge of the distal nail plate. "Pitting of the fingernails with lifting and flaring is supportive of the diagnosis of psoriasis, and a change suggestive of an oil droplet underneath the nail is pathognomonic." This quotation, from *Cecil's Textbook of Medicine* (1992), emphasises the importance of fingernail examination in psoriasis. This disorder may begin at any age, but occurs more usually in young adults. The peak incidence is in people in their 30s. HLA tissue typing markers are useful only in determining whether there is some inherited component. Patients with HL-A$_{13}$ tissue type have a milder form of the disease and little heritable tendency, whereas W$_{17}$ patients have a significant number of affected relatives and an earlier age of onset.

Psoriasishas no specific known cure, but remissions which were previously seasonal can be enhanced by using combinations of various tar preparations and ultraviolet light. The fingernails may be affected before there are widespread generalised lesions, although small lesions can be found in the region of the elbows or knees in 95% of patients with definite psoriatic changes in the nails. In a few unusual cases, the nail changes are said to antedate the more generalised skin changes by up to several years. Well-documented cases are rare.

Typical Nail Plate Changes

Reliable studies on the histology show that increasing nail involvement, especially of the matrix cells, leads to an irregular, dirty, mottled appearance, increasing onycholysis spreading towards the cuticle and matrix area and, eventually, the shedding of the nail itself. With such appearances and in more severe cases, the terminal joints may also be affected. In moderate psoriasis of the skin, 50% of patients will have nail changes.

Destructive Psoriasis

Cells starting from the basal level of the nails take 3–4 days to reach the surface layers in psoriatic nails, whereas in normal nails, the time scale is 3–4 weeks. Migration and normal keratinisation do not have time to take place evenly, especially if the psoriasis is patchy. Thus, rapid progress of cells reaching the surface in psoriatic zones mean that cells still have their nucleus and become parakeratotic. Sometimes the shedding is incomplete and patchy. This may allow infection, and micro-abscesses filled with polymorpholeucocytes are seen in examples of the so-called pustular psoriatic nails. Eventually, exuberant activity of the basal cells takes place with coarse thickening and overgrowth of the misshapen nails.

References

1. Dawber, R. Fingernail growth in normal and psoriatic subjects. *British Journal of Dermatology,* 1970, **82**, 454.
2. Dawber, R., Samman, P. D. & Bottoms, E. Fingernail growth in idiopathic and psoriatic onycholysis. *British Journal of Dermatology,* 1971, **85**, 558.
3. Farber, E. M. & Nall, L. Nail psoriasis. *Cutis,* 1992, **50** (3), 174–8.
4. Grassi, W., Core, P., Carlino, G., & Cervini, C. Nailfold capillary permeability in psoriatic arthritis. *Scandinavian Journal of Rheumatology,* 1992, **21** (5), 226–30.
5. Lewin, K., Dewit, S. & Ferrington, R. A. Pathology of the finger nail in psoriasis. *British Journal of Dermatology*, 1972, **86**, 555.
6. Leyden, J. J. Exfoliate cytology in the diagnosis of psoriasis of the nails. *Cutis,* 1972, **10**, 701.
7. Rothenberg, S., Crounse, R. G. & Lee, J. L. Glycine–C14 incorporation into the proteins of normal stratum corneum and the abnormal stratum corneum of psoriasis. *Journal of Investigative Dermatology and Syph.,* 1961, **37**, 497.
8. Rudolph, R. I. Lithium-induced psoriasis of the fingernails. *Journal of the American Academy of Dermatology,* 1992, **26** (1), 135–6.
9. Trevisan, G., Magaton Rizzi, G. & Dal Canton, M. Psoriatic microangiopathy modifications induced by PUVA and etretinate therapy. A nail-fold capillary microscopic study. *Acta Dermato-Venereologica Suppl.* (Stockholm), 1989, **146**, 53–6.

Minimal Nail Changes

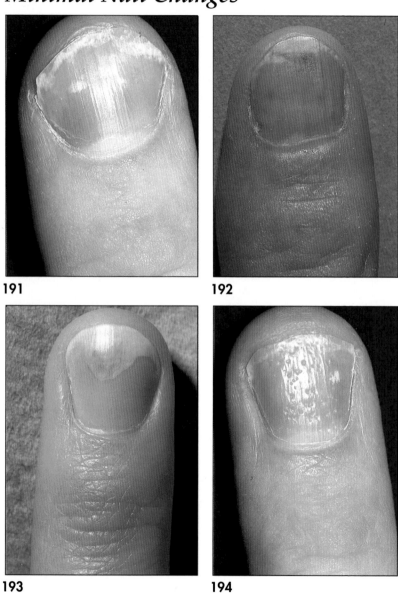

191

192

193

194

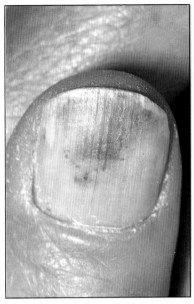

195

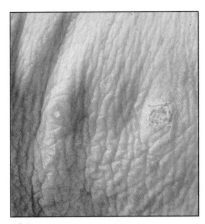

196

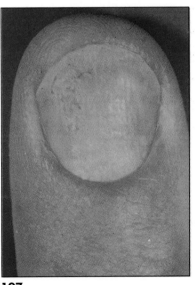

197

191 Very mild psoriasis. Minimal changes in the free margin of the nail of a woman in her 30s.

192 Discolouration and distal lysis in the nail of a young Maori male experiencing minimal nail plate changes.

193 Psoriasis of nail producing only localised lysis (young woman).

194 Minimal skin changes in this woman who showed "Roseneau" pitting of nails and later developed psoriasis on her elbows.

195 Minimal pitting but marked discolouration in a psoriatic nail.

196 Elbow lesion of psoriasis. This was the first lesion to develop 2 years after onycholysis seen in **204** (page 127).

197 Minimal skin changes but all nails involved. Opacity and flaking of all nail surface in psoriasis.

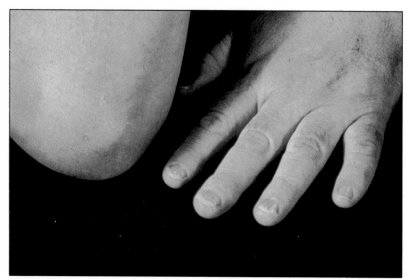

198

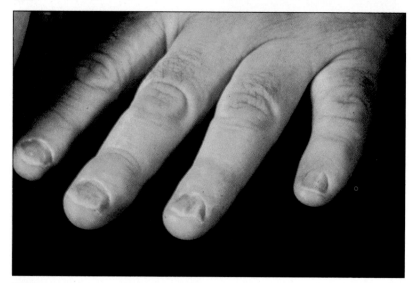

199

Typical Nail Changes in Psoriasis

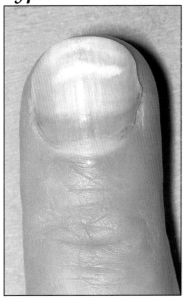

200

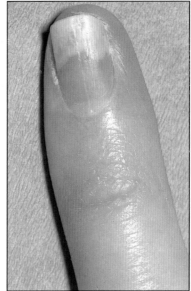

201

198 Elbow–knee syndrome in psoriasis.
199 Hand with nail involvement. Elbow–knee syndrome in psoriasis.
200 Interesting half-nail lysis to give leukonychia.
201 Nail lysis in psoriasis with evidence of minimal skin changes over knuckle.

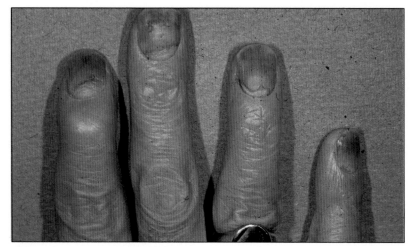

202

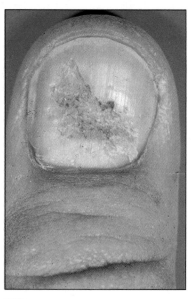

203

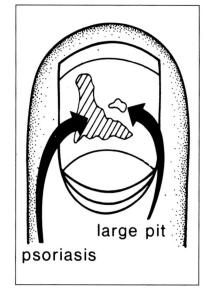

large pit

psoriasis

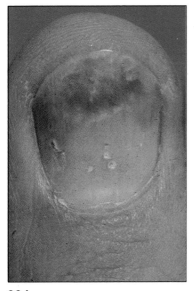

204

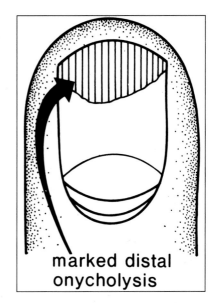

marked distal onycholysis

202 Typical advanced changes could almost be mistaken for yellow-nail syndrome. This elderly woman also has marked distal psoriatic arthropathy.

203 Central nail plate involved. Diffuse psoriatic skin condition with diffuse but mild dystrophia shown on most of the nails.

204 Onycholysis antedating skin lesion. Early distal onycholysis led to consultation with many doctors. Eventually, a small lesion on the left elbow led to the correct diagnosis of psoriatic nail disease.

205 Differential diagnosis. Nail dystrophy in a middle-aged woman. This is secondary to a generalised dermatitis, thought to be drug-induced and now healed. Psoriasis questioned.

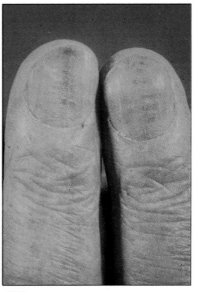

205

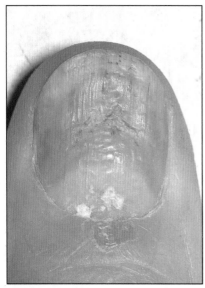

206

206 Multiple changes with terminal and lateral lysis, nail plate changes (pseudo-Leclercq) and active skin disease.

207 Marked thickening of fingernails in chronic and difficult psoriasis.

208 Severely affected and destroyed nails from unremitting and chronic psoriasis. Also marked arthropathy.

209 Destructive pustular psoriasis.

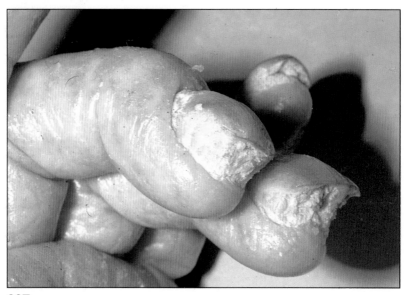

207

Destructive Nail Changes

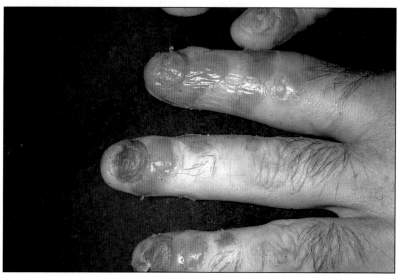

208

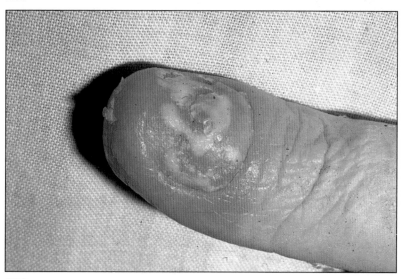

209

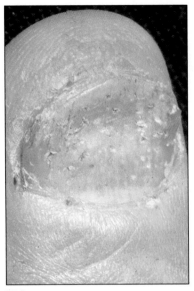
210

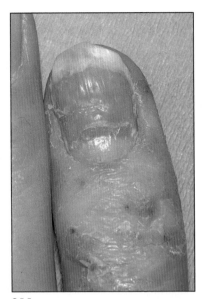
211

210 Destructive effects minimised by shortened "nail".
211 Destructive effect on nail limited to 5th digit nail. Now in quiescent phase.

Chapter 10
Clubbing of Fingers & Fingernails

Fingernail clubbing is one of the most widely known signs of general systemic disease. Indeed, it was the great Greek physician Hippocrates who described clubbing of the fingernails in a patient with empyema in the fifth century BC. To the primary care physician or general internist, the earliest definite signs of clubbing are usually an important signal of the presence of lung, heart or gastrointestinal disease.

A proposed method of "rocking" the nail plate has been reliably used by one of the authors over two decades, and is well illustrated here. Various forms of grading of the degrees of severity are preferable to the separate names sometimes used for more severe degrees (such as hypertrophic pulmonary arthropathy).

What causes clubbing? Editorials in the *Lancet* and *British Medical Journal* testify to its importance, and yet the exact mechanism by which excess growth of the matrix cells is stimulated is not fully known. The best current hypothesis to fit in with known facts is that there is a combination of autonomic nerve control of the digital arterioles, together with changes in the ratio of circulating vaso-active kinins perfusing the finger pulp. Some of the blood supply carrying nutrients to the proximal nail bed and matrix passes through the very active fingertip plexus in the termal pulp.Well-recognised "capillary shunts" here are opened and shut according to the need to lose or conserve heat. Thus, in pulmonary causes of clubbing, such as obstruction and then dilatation of the bronchi, autonomic stimulus will play a major role; whereas in cyanotic heart disease or liver disease, changes in the vaso-active peptides could divert more stimulated blood to the nail bed.

A common list of causes of "simple" clubbing is set out to emphasise the value of observing early clubbing in systemic disease (*see Table 3, p. 133*). Other more specific types of clubbing which are given a separate classification are hypertrophic osteoarthropathy and pachydermoperiostitis. The former, usually seen in rapidly growing cancer of the lung or bronchus, is really pseudo-inflammatory but is also associated with pseudoarthropathies. The latter is a rarer version of hypertrophic osteoarthropathy where a line of periosteal new bone is lifted up and can be seen on x-rays of the tips of the fingers or toes. A further sub-classification of clubbing is sometimes called the "shell-nail" syndrome, in which some long-standing bronchiectatic patients develop thin, clubbed nails with atrophy of the underlying bone and nail bed.

"Clawing" of the fingertips is characteristic of long-term smokers—particularly in women. Here the pulp becomes wasted and the nail curved over but with no filling in of the proximal nail fold and no easy rockability. As the patient gradually develops increasing degrees of lung failure due to panacinar emphysema, the fingernails become more and more curved. With the loss of pulp, the fingertips come to resemble talons. In the early stages this goes by the name of "beaking", as the nails curve to resemble a bird's beak; when the curving of the nails later becomes more pronounced, assuming a claw-like appearance, they are described as "claw nails". The condition is referred to either as "clawing" or "beaking". The loss of digital pulp or lack of pulp growth distinguishes clawing from clubbing.

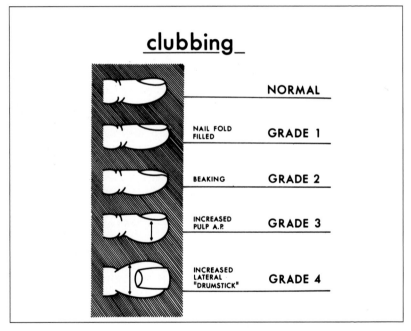

212

212   Grading of finger nail clubbing.

TABLE 3.

Commoner Causes of Clubbing

Bilateral and also Toes

- Pulmonary from any obstruction causing dilatation to tracheal or bronchial branches.
- Cardiovascular (usually of cyanotic heart disease or valvular origin).
- Gastrointestinal:
  - Diffuse liver disease.
  - Inflammatory bowel disease, with or without diverticulae.
  - Tropical sprue.
  - Small gut disease.
  - Chronic gut parasites.
- Metabolic—usually malnutrition, rarely in hypothyroidism.
- Congenital and usually familial.

Unilateral

- Aortic or subclavian artery aneurysm..
- Autonomic involvement in brachial plexus injury.

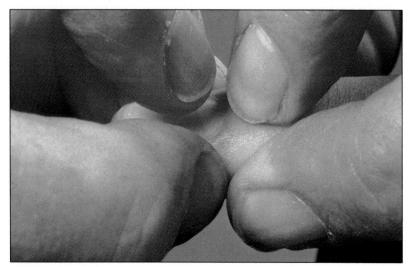

213

213 & 214   Method for demonstrating "rocking". When Grade 1 or early clubbing occurs, the first sign is a filling in of the nail fold with loss of angle. This area immediately over the nail fold or matrix becomes spongy. The front and back halves of the nail may be "rocked" as in a see-saw. This may be achieved by gripping the sides of the nails between the thumb and middle finger of each hand. The two index fingers can then rock the nail up and down. Part of the see-saw is depressed with the left index finger (**213**). Then the left index finger is lifted and the right index finger depresses the most proximal end of the nail over the matrix and under the nail fold (**214**). These movements are repeated to develop a sensation of rocking with the rapidly growing nail matrix under the nail plate as the fulcrum.

215   Measuring clubbing by x-ray. Standardised method of measuring angle and degree of clubbing from a lateral radiograph of the finger.

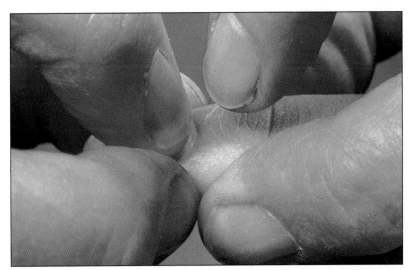

214

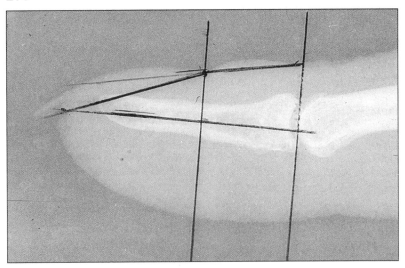

215

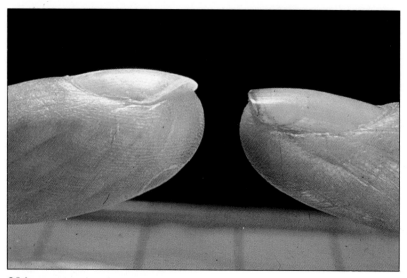

216

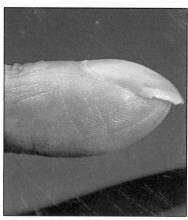

217

216 Early clubbing. Early clubbing (Grade 2) in a young woman with single lobe bronchiectasis. Comparison with age matched control (on right).

217 Rapid onset clubbing. Grade 2 clubbing in a middle-aged man with fibrosing alveolitis of some duration.

218 Clubbing and other findings. Early clubbing in patient with subacute bacterial endocarditis. This man is also a smoker; note nicotine staining. Two small "splinter" haemorrhages are also present.

219 Clubbing and pigmentation. Marked clubbing of nail in an elderly male with chronic lung disease and some bronchiectasis in a collapsed middle lobe. Also has lung failure with hypoxia. This latter appears to be the only cause of the increasing pigmentation.

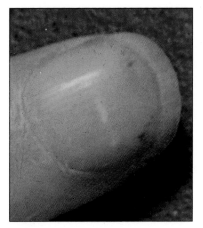

218

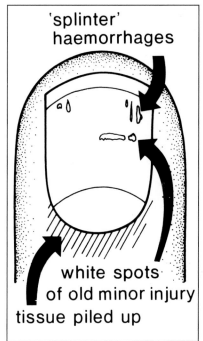

'splinter' haemorrhages

white spots
of old minor injury
tissue piled up

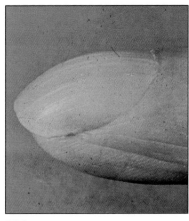

219

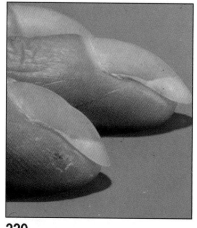

220

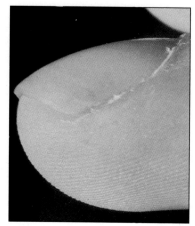

221

220 Clubbing with cyanosis. This elderly railway worker presented with cough and sputum. Note clubbing, some beaking and pulp wasting of middle finger, suggesting chronic hypoxia. Also, marked cyanosis indicative of unsaturated haemoglobin, either due to polycythaemia compensatory to the long-term low oxygen levels or to severe blood gas mismatch problems. Lung abscess present.

221 Clubbing in younger person. More severe clubbing in long-standing bronchiectasis. Note also aneamia and marked increase in sponginess at inner nail fold. Fluctuation of the nail bed is apparent at this site.

222 Immediate diagnosis in a 72-year-old labourer who was a life-long smoker. Note strongly positive "nicotine sign". Presented with painful fingertips. Gross drumstick Grade 4 clubbing of nails and x-ray confirmed an inoperable bronchogenic cancer of the lung.

223 "Intestinal clubbing". Gross clubbing (Grade 4) in a 42-year-old man who developed tropical sprue while serving in the army—with continuing diarrhoea and several bone fractures. Found to have low levels of serum calcium and phosphorus, with x-ray appearances of osteomalacia in the bones. Tests and small gut biopsy confirmed malabsorption due to small gut disease. Normal lungs, cardiovascular system and liver function.

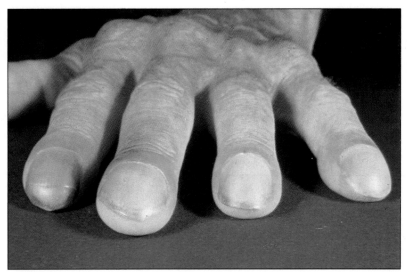

222

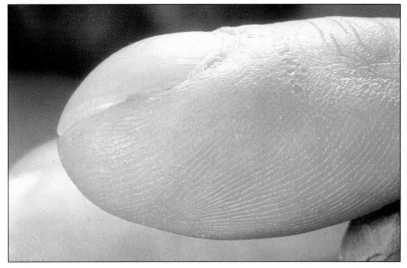

223

139

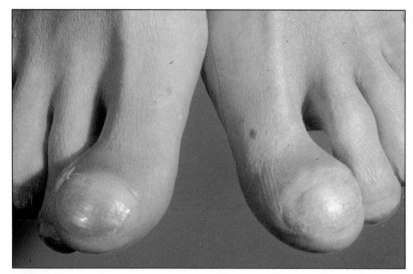

224

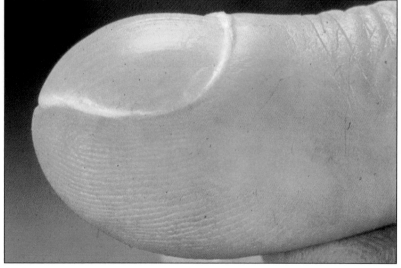

225

140

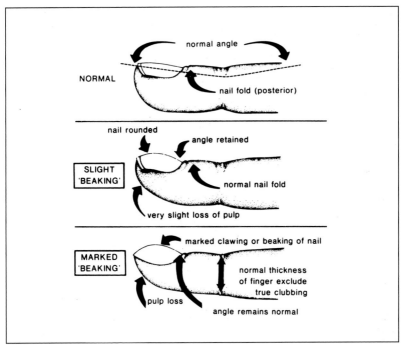

226

224 Toes are clubbed as well. Clubbing when well marked in Grades 3 or 4 is also observed in all the toes of this woman with chronic lung disease and bronchiectasis.
225 Another gut disease. Gross (Grade 4) clubbing in small gut disease.
226 Beaking of the nails.

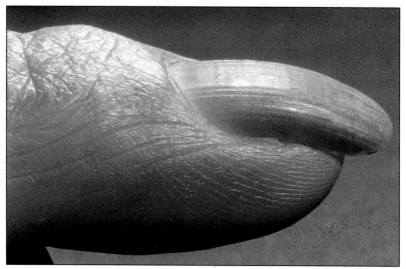

227

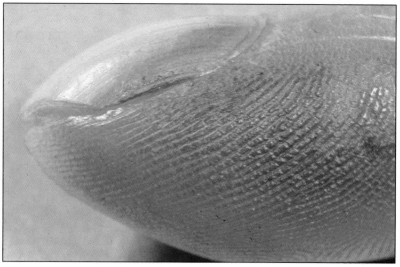

228

142

227 "Beaking" or "clawing". Marked nicotine staining in an elderly, retired wire worker who remained addicted to smoking although experiencing gradual loss of lung tissue due to obstructive airways disease and emphysema. Note thickening and dystrophy of nail secondary to previous occupational trauma, beaking and pulp.

228 "Beaking or "clawing". Severe beaking of nails in a heavy smoker with hypoxia (pAO_2 = 55) and lung x-rays showing only emphysema with obstructive lung disease.

References

1. Leading article. Finger clubbing and hypertrophic pulmonary osteoarthropathy. *British Medical Journal*, 1977, **3**, 785.
2. *The Genuine Works of Hippocrates*. Translated by Adams, F. V. 1849, **1**, 249.
3. Leading article. Finger clubbing. *Lancet,* 1975, **i**, 1285.
4. Ponchon, Y., Chelloul, N. & Roujeau, J. Contribution a l'etude anatamopathologique de l'hippocratisme digital. *Semaine des Hopitaux de Paris,* 1969, **42**, 2604.
5. Racoceanu, S. M., Mendlowitz, M., Suck, A. F., Wolf, R. L. & Naftchi, N. E. *Annals of Internal Medicine,* 1971, **75**, 933.
6. Stone, O. J. & Maberry, J. D. Spoon nails and clubbing. Review and possible mechanisms. *Texas State Journal of Medicine,* 1965, **61**, 620.
7. Young, J. R. Ulcerative colitis and finger clubbing. *British Medical Journal,* 1966, **1**, 278.

Chapter 11
Nail Changes Seen in General Medical Conditions

During the last decade there has been a resurgence of interest in a quick scrutiny of the fingernails after introduction to a new patient or client. The primary care doctor or health worker has immediate access to the observation of 10 fingernails as part of the physical examination.

This routine examination of the nails should always be carried out within the framework and as part of the normal physical examination. As a method for eliciting information and as a means of teaching deductions from observations, it is much more useful than pulse taking. Because it reflects past and present health, it allows a wider and more varied series of deductions, including those from the skin and integument, state of nutrition and health, attitudes, personality and occupation.

In over a thousand consecutive admissions of patients over the age of 60 to the general medical ward of a teaching hospital, seldom did examination of the fingernails fail to reveal valuable information about a person's make-up and background. Furthermore, 28% had markedly abnormal changes in the nails, useful for both the teaching of trainee doctors and as a source of additional data about the systemic disorders present. Many older patients have abnormalities of the nails such as those described in other chapters— Beau's lines, koilonychia, clubbing, loss of lunula due to low serum albumen, and other interesting signs including changes in the nail plate, shape or colour of the nails. Collagen disorders such as scleroderma and dermatomyositis may result in significant nail changes. The following group of nails emphasises the wide variety of general medical disorders from splinter haemorrhages (Miller & Vaziri, 1979) to thyrotoxicosis and Addison's disease, which may result in characteristic changes in the nails.

If, during the normal examination, any abnormality of the nail is seen, a cause or explanation should be sought. So often, elderly patients who have slowly developing nutritional deficiencies may accept as the normal evolution of old age such changes which are clearly abnormal to a trained observer. The real tragedy is if their primary care physician does the same, which may occur either because of a failure to make the correct deductions from the right observations, or a failure to examine the nails. Nothing is more encouraging to both the doctor or health worker and patient than a wide range of correct deductions being made in the first minutes of clinical examination or greeting.

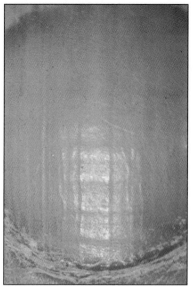

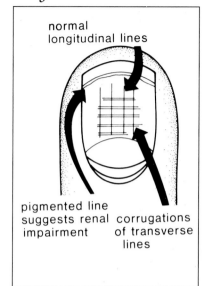

229

229 Repeated illness. This thumbnail comes from a 67-year-old man with repeated severe Stokes-Adams attacks.

230 Valuable nail signs. Index fingernail of a 76-year-old widow with chronic and repeated episodes of left ventricular failure. She had become depressed, as manifested by the poor manicure at the base of the nail and the nails were slightly cyanosed. Warm skin temperature on handshake suggests this is central cyanosis and suggests some pulmonary oedema at the lung bases. The flattened front half of the nails may also suggest poor diet, which was indeed the case because of digoxin toxity. Note also lack of lunula and some "beading" in the normal longitudinal ridges of the nails.

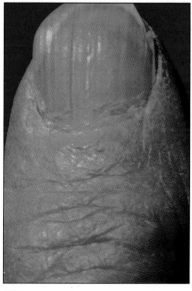

230

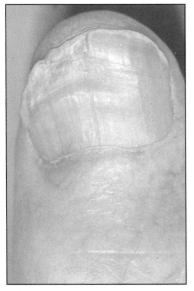

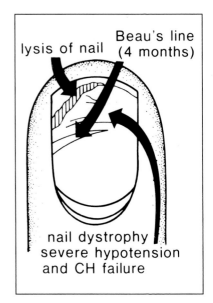

lysis of nail

Beau's line (4 months)

nail dystrophy
severe hypotension
and CH failure

231

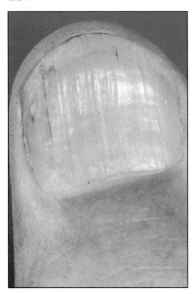

232

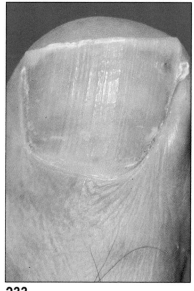

233

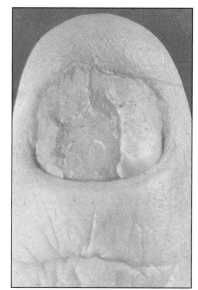

234

231 Useful signs. Thumbnail from 73-year-old non–insulin-dependent diabetic male who 8 months previously had suffered myocardial infarction with poor output and hypotension. Note onycholysis on the leading edge and 1–2 months of dystrophic growth. Then a further infarction (4-month-old Beau's line). Also long-standing diabetic proteinuria and lowered serum albumen.

232 Widespread atheroma. The thumbnail of a 79-year-old male with onset of left middle cerebral artery thrombosis. Beau's lines and longitudinal ridges can be seen; left and right sides show markedly similar changes.

233 Beading toenail. Great toenail from 73-year-old non–insulin-dependent man with repeated heart trouble.

234 Nail shedding secondary to atheroma. An elderly male with gross aortic arch atheroma and ischaemia in hand.

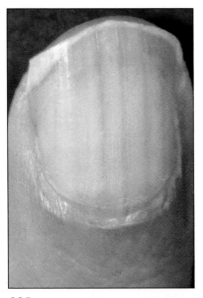
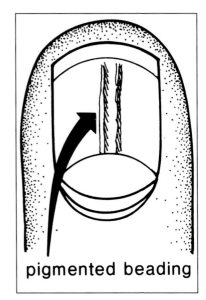

pigmented beading

235

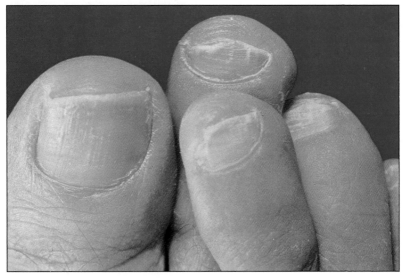

236

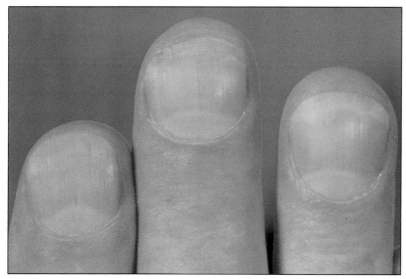

237

235 and 236 Pigmented beading. Thumbnail and toenails of a 35-year-old woman. These are from the right side of the body of a patient who had a hemispherectomy 25 years ago. Note pigmented longitudinal ridges in thumb and spasticity of toes.

237 Chronic left heart failure. Fingernails of a 77-year-old retired accountant with chronic left ventricular failure. Note excellent lunula, bluish nails, early onycholysis and "heaped up" posterior nail fold.

238 Severe Raynaud's. Very severe Raynaud's phenomenon in feet with failure to respond to treatment. Secondary to autoimmune disease—note changes in skin colour.

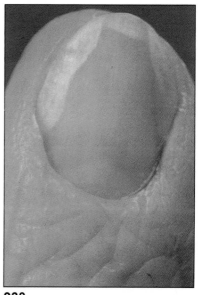

238

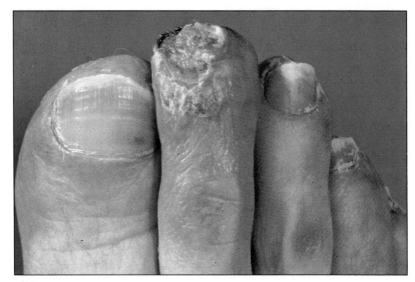

239

239 Raynaud's disease. Arrow-shaped nails resulting from lateral onycholysis in elderly woman with long-term Raynaud's disease.
240–243 Photographs of nails of patient with renal failure and hyperparathyroidism, showing terminal bone absorption in the last digit of each finger.

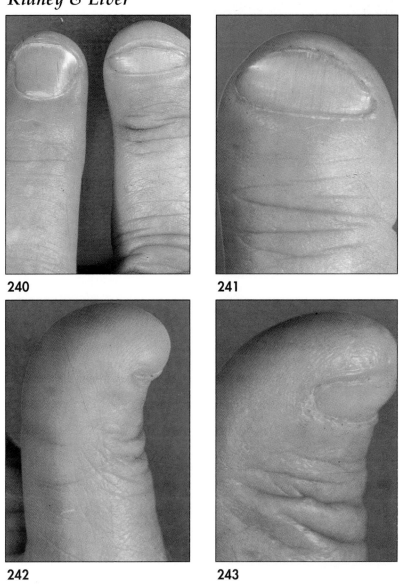

240

241

242

243

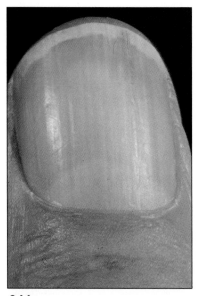

244

244 Early kidney failure. Interesting thumbnails of a 38-year-old Caucasian woman with a 27-year history of diabetes, now slowly developing renal failure.

245 Multiple changes in kidney failure. Middle-aged woman with progressive renal failure and rising blood urea. Poor appetite has led to some malnutritional changes with koilonychia and loss of lunula. Pigment below yellow line also seen in kidney failure and some early onycholysis of nutritional origin.

246 Maori boy with kidney failure. Thumbnail of a 15-year-old boy who had a renal transplant one month previously. Note marked growth arrest line and pigmentation at base of nail.

247 Liver damage. Fingers from woman with alcohol liver disease. Note infection and increased blood flow at base of nail. Also loss of lunula and onycholysis.

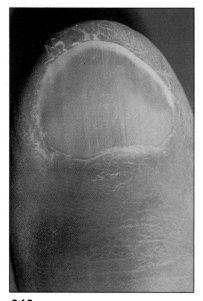

245

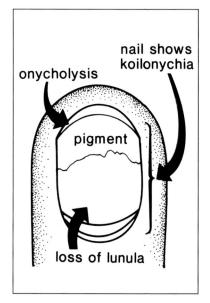

152

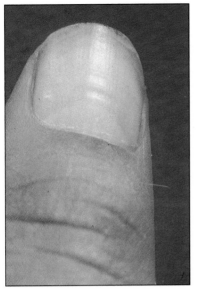

246

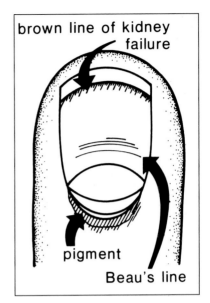

brown line of kidney failure

pigment

Beau's line

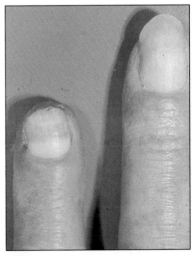

247

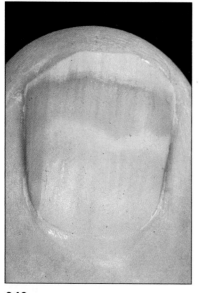

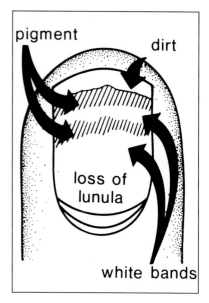

248

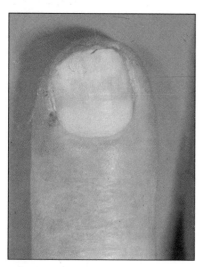

249

248 Muehrck's white bands. Liver disease and early cirrhosis in a 38-year-old alcoholic woman showing loss of lunula and white bands. Serum albumen at lower limit of normal.

249 Terry's half-and-half nail. From same middle-aged woman with alcoholic liver disease and low serum albumen.

250 Pancreatic damage. Diabetes in a middle-aged lawyer. Pale nails and poorly defined lunula but serum albumen normal.

251 Nutritional. General nail dystrophy in middle-aged woman with upper gastro-intestinal disease. Note lateral onycholysis, opacity and granularity of nail. Lunula is reduced. Poor manicure due to chronic ill health.

252 Acromegalic fingers in both hands.

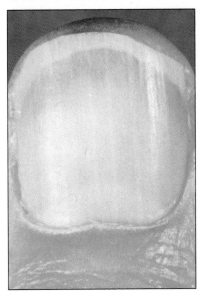

250

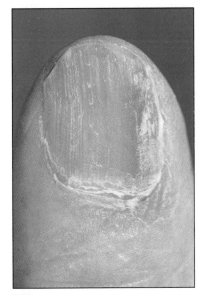

251

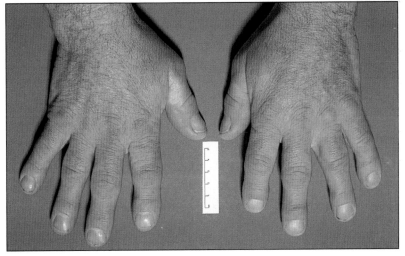

252

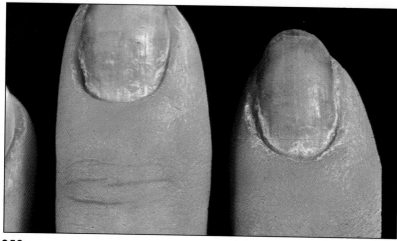

253

253 Acromegalic fingers. Untreated acromegaly in a 32-year-old school teacher with chronic fungus infection in middle and index fingernails. Note statistical association between acromegaly with carbohydrate intolerance and high incidence of fungal infection of nails.

254 Acquired brachyonchia. Characteristic shrinking of terminal phalanx in secondary hyperparathyroidism.

255 Elderly thyrotoxic. Thumbnail of hospitalised 80-year-old woman with congestive heart failure on basis of thyrotoxicosis. Note change in skin, good lunula, pigment in skin at nail base and beading present in the longitudinal ridges usually seen in patients of this age.

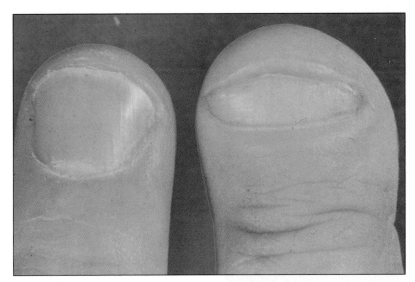

254

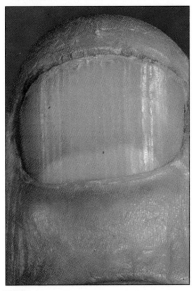

255

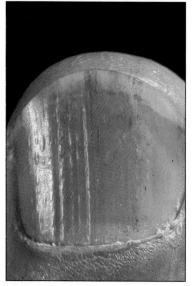

256

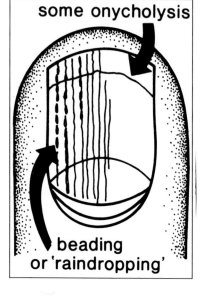

some onycholysis

beading
or 'raindropping'

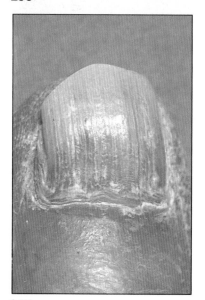

257

256 Thyrotoxicosis. Marked beading or "raindropping" in an elderly thyrotoxic male. Picture at diagnosis. Also called "sausaging".

257 Middle-aged salesman presenting with long-standing Cushing's syndrome and reduced immunity status.

258 and 259 Toes of a 67-year-old newly diagnosed diabetic man on a small dose of prednisolone for asthma. Note bifid toes, a small callus on one toe and marked fungal infection in the nail of the adjacent toe. More than half of all toenails were affected.

Diabetes Mellitus

Diabetes mellitus affects 3–4% of adult populations in most countries around the world. The complications of the hyperglycaemic and hyperlipidaemia are frequently seen in outpatient's clinics, general practice and in hospital beds. Long-standing diabetes is often the cause of koilonychia, commonly seen in the fingernails of men with this condition (*see Chapter 3*), and may also lead to renal failure if poorly controlled.

Insulin and growth hormone are necessary for transport across the matrix cell wall of sulphur-containing amino-acids and their subsequent incorporation into the specialised nail plate. As leukocytes fail in both phagocytosis and immunity functions in insulin deficiency states, fungal infections are commonly seen in the nails of those with diabetes, particularly in the toenails, where ischaemia from large and small blood vessel disease compounds the problem of immune failure. The feet and toenails are also affected, either from critical ischaemia with the threat of "dry" or infected gangrene or from neuropathy. Examples of some of these conditions may be seen in the following illustrations.

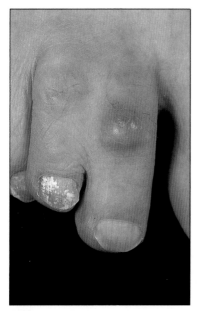

258

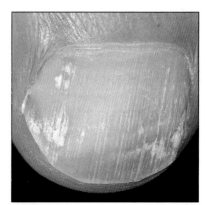

259

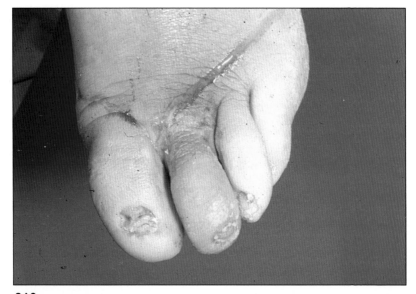

260

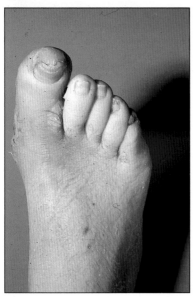

261

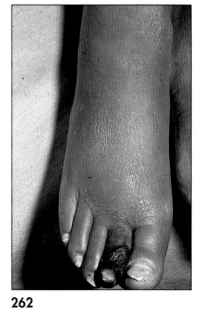

262

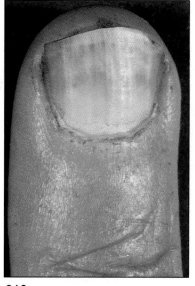

263

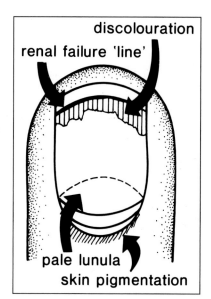

discolouration
renal failure 'line'
pale lunula
skin pigmentation

260 Foot of 72-year-old man with long-standing diabetes, thickening of the skin and so-called "dry" gangrene. Viltration sense was measured to be only 20% of normal, and pulses were absent.

261 The cold foot and toes show atrophic scaling skin changes and lack of sensation due to neuropathy, compounded by more critical recent ischaemia.

262 The toenail of an elderly Polynesian man was infected with fungus and was lost when the toe was amputated. He had an acute secondary bacterial infection affecting the web space of the foot.

263 Diabetic kidney failure. Finger of a 47-year-old man with insulin-dependent diabetes of 22 years' duration. Early visual failure due to retinopathy (note poor manicure) and protein-losing nephropathy; blood urea also raised.

264 Infection under the great toenail of an elderly diabetic man, now in end stage of healing. Note colour due to ischaemic fungal infection in 2nd toe.

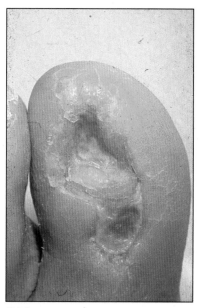

264

Scleroderma, Dermatomyosis & Autoimmune Disease

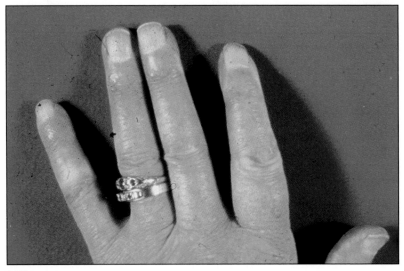

265

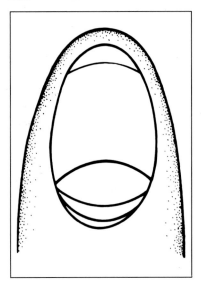

265 Scleroderma hands. Nails taper to a point with tethering of tissue in scleroderma.

266 Scleroderma. 41-year-old man with scleroderma presenting as early renal failure. Note extreme ridging of nail, poor manicure and loss of lunula. Tips of digits are narrowed.

267 Extrusion under nail. Nails of an elderly woman with severe scleroderma.

268 Middle-aged woman with fairly acute onset of dermatomyosis, skin lesions near nails and raised muscle enzymes.

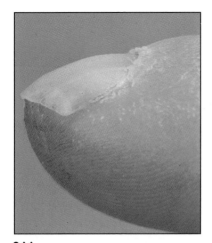

266

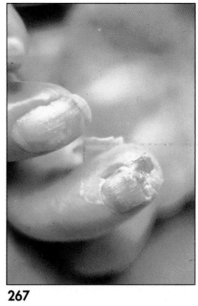

267

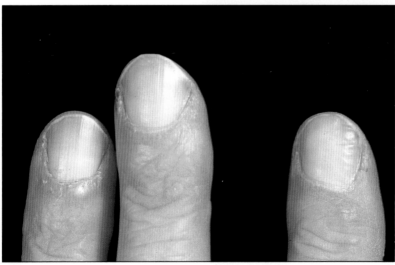

268

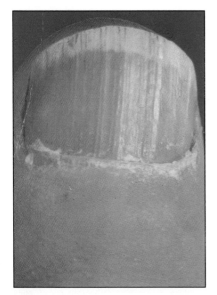

269

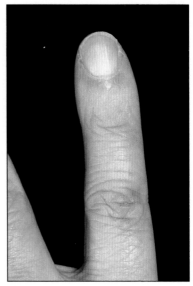

270

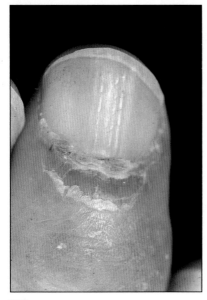

271

164

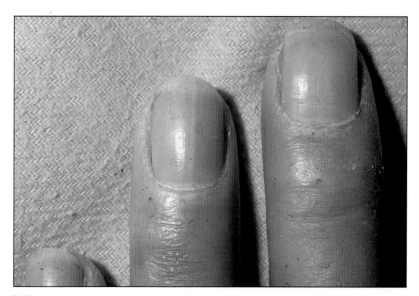

272

269   Scleroderma and renal failure. Non-specific ridges but also loss of lunula and poor manicure.

270   Closer view of affected finger and nail of same patient as in **295** (Chapter 12, page 176). Some impairment of renal function—see free edge nail.

271   Periungual vasculitis in a middle-aged (44-year-old) woman with acute onset rheumatoid arthritis and autoimmune markers.

272   *Lupus erythematosus* nail fold erythoma.

Blood & General

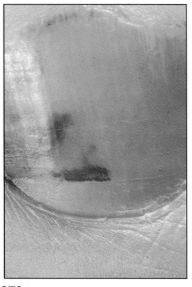

273 Bleeding under nail. Butazolidin-induced thrombotic thrombocytopenic purpura in a 70-year-old farmer being treated for arthritis of the hip.

274 Close-up of subungual distal haemorrhages. Note bleeding in distal nail bed, which suggests spontaneous occurrence.

275 Koilonychia with developing median splitting, thickened nail and hyperkeratosis of skin in 63-year-old man with chronic leukaemia.

276 Subungual haemorrhages. Elderly male with lymphoblastic stage of acute or chronic leukaemia. Subungual-induced low platelets. Note also ground-glass appearance of the rest of the nail.

273

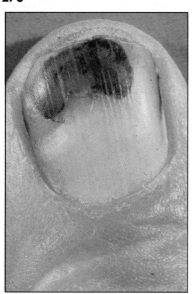

274

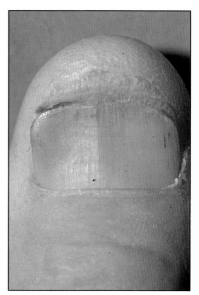

275

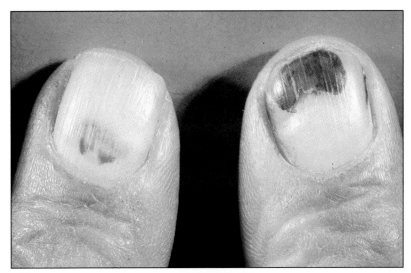

276

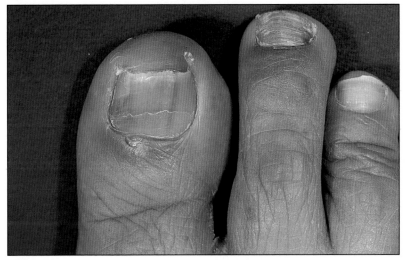

277

277 Pigmented streaks, transverse stria and fungal infections in an African with proven Burkitt's lymphoma—referred to exudate a secondary malignant subungual melanoma.

References

1. Ames, D. E., Asherson, R. A., Ayres, B., Cassar J. & Hughes, G. R. Bilateral adrenal infarction, hypoadrenalism and splinter haemorrhages in the 'primary'antiphospholipid syndrome. *British Journal of Rheumatology,* 1992, **31** (2), 117–120.

2. Dalziel, K. L., Telfer, N. R. & Dawber, R. P. Nail dystrophy in cutaneous T–cell lymphoma. *British Journal of Dermatology,* 1989, **120** (4), 571–574.

3. Diven, D. G., Gwinup, G., Newton, R. C. The thyroid. *Dermatol. Clin.,* 1989, **7** (3), 547–558.

4. Gertner, E., Sukenik, S., Gladman, D. D., Hanna, W., Lee, P., Bombardier, C., Hanna, A. K. HLA antigens and nailfold capillary microscopy studies in patients with insulin-dependent and non–insulin-dependent diabetes mellitus and limited joint mobility. *J. Rheumatol.,* 1990, **17** (10), 1375–1379.

5. Gross, N. J. & Tall, R. Clinical significance of splinter haemorrhages. *British Medical Journal,* 1963, 2, 1496.

6. Hamilton, E. D. B. Nail studies in rheumatoid arthritis. *Annals of Rheumatic Diseases,* 1960, **19**, 167.

7. Held, J. L, Chew, S., Grossman, M. E. & Kohn, S. R. Transverse striate leukonychia associated with acute rejection of renal allograft. *Journal of the American Academy of Dermatologists,* 1989, **20** (3), 513–514.

8. Leyden, J. J. & Wood, M. F. The half and half nail of uremic onychodystrophy. *Archives of Dermatology,* 1972, **105**, 591.

9. Miller, A. & Vaziri, N. D. Recurrent traumatic subungual splinter haemorrhages in healthy individuals. *South African Medical Journal,* 1979, **72** (11), 1418.

10. Norton, L. A. Nail disorders. A review. *Journal of the American Academy of Dermatologists,* 1980, **2** (6), 451.

11. Quenneville, J. G. & Gossard, D. Subungual–splinter haemorrhage: an early sign of thromboangitis obliterans. *American Journal of Diseases of Childhood,* 1981, **135** (4). 383.

12. Ridley, C. M. Pigmentation of fingertips and nails in vitamin B_{12} deficiency. *British Journal of Dermatology,* 1977, **97** (1),105.

13. Saner, H. E., Wurbel, H., Gurtner, H. P. & Mahler, F. Increased peripheral vasoconstrictor reaction upon local cold in patients with coronary heart disease. *Int. J. Microcirc. Clin. Exp.,* 1989, **8** (2), 127–34.

14. Ulowitz, M. B., Gladman, D. D., Chalmers, A. & Ogryzlo, M. A. Nail lesions in systemic lupus erythematous. *Journal of Rheumatology,* 1978, **5** (4), 441.

15. Verra, F., Kouzan, S., Saig, P., Bigon, J. & de Cremoux, H. Bronchioalveolar disease in dyskeratosis congenita. *European Respiratory Journal,* 1992, **5** (4), 497–9.

Chapter 12
Nail Changes Associated with Intellectual Disability & Congenital Disorders

It is increasingly accepted that nail abnormalities may be part of a more general syndrome resulting from an isolated chromosome defect or part of a more general inherited abnormality. A history of any abnormal maternal exposure to drugs or illness during pregnancy is often helpful.

Monosomia 4, 7 & 9, trisomy 9, 13, 21, & X and quadrosomy X have all been described in association with nail changes, and brachyonychia, (short nails), micronychia, nail en racquette, lack of lunula, fused nails and syndactyly are all unusual and rare findings which indicate a clear need for careful family history and specialised chromosome analysis. Increasingly, DNA probes will be used.

A wide range of autosomal recessive and dominant syndromes can be associated with short broad nails. This short, abnormal end digit, with often broad thumbs, frequently has associated skeletal changes in the jaws and skull. Attention may be drawn to this because of "pseudo-clubbing" or other nail or teeth abnormalities (various ectodermal dysplasia syndromes).

The most commonly seen of the multitude of such rare syndromes are:
- Nail-patella syndrome (chromosome 9);
- Sézary syndrome;
- Rubinstein–Taybi syndrome;
- Various dyskeratoses; or
- Hair–nail dysplasia.

Thus, very many other rare syndromes may be brought to attention by nail "markers". Examples of these include the following:
- Autosomal dominant—i.e. ectodermal dysplasias with onychic subgroups.
- Inherited and familial metabolic disorders—i.e. homocystinuria.
- Specific chromosomal abnormalities—i.e. trisomy 21 with micromychia, incurving 5th finger, etc. (Down's syndrome and variants).
- Normal, known karyotype, but hereditary disorders—i.e. Apert's syndrome (fused digits and nails).
- X-linked disorders usually recessive—i.e. syndromes with broad, short nails, bone hypoplasia, cleft palate, etc.

169

Down's syndrome (Trisomy 21)

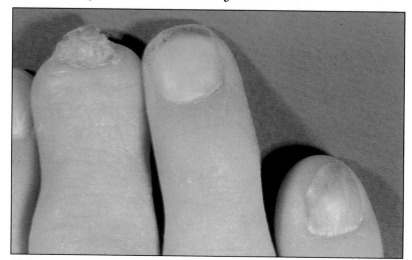

278

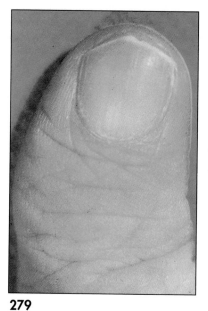

279

280

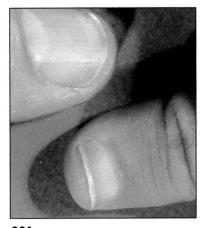

281

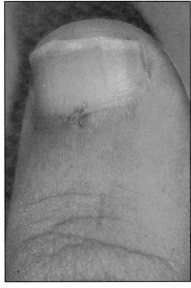

282

278 Trisomy 21 in adult patient of moderate intellectual impairment. Minimal degree of psoriasis also present with right 5th finger affected. Left 5th finger shows normal Down's sydnrome features; incurving of finger with reduced lunula, convexity and increased longitudinal ridges. As well as psoriasis, the middle finger also shows an old injury.

279 Trisomy 21. Incurving 5th finger. Poor nail cutting and absent lunula.

280 "Old" nail for 18 years. Incurving short 5th finger as seen in trisomy 21. Note that the nail is also abnormally narrow with longitudinal ridges.

281 Common brachyonychia (bottom finger). Usual micronychia in trisomy 21 in normal adult of the same age for comparison (top finger).

282 Brachyonychia thumb. Trisomy 21 with profound mental disability. Note micronychia of thumbnail. No epicanthic fold changes, but marked laxity of ligaments.

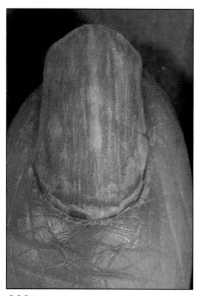

283

283 and 284 Nail dystrophy. Trisomy 21 with unilateral arm, oedema and marked nail dystrophy. Other side shows usual appearances in Down's syndrome with short thumbnail and incurving 5th finger. On unaffected side, poor development of the lunula is visible.

285 Down's syndrome. Short nail, abnormally convex, lacking lunula.

286 Trisomy 21, Down's syndrome. Thumbnail within normal limits, whereas often short in Down's syndrome.

287 Trisomy 21—5th finger. Nails typical of Down's syndrome. Note incurving 5th finger with short, broad nail, which also shows micro-onychia and loss of lunula.

288 Probable trisomy 21. Microcephaly and severe mental disability. Nail dysplasia and lysis. No chromosome studies yet available.

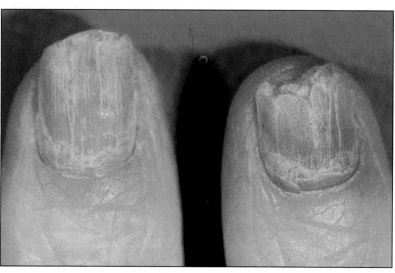

284

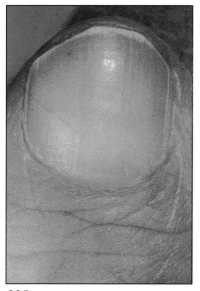

285

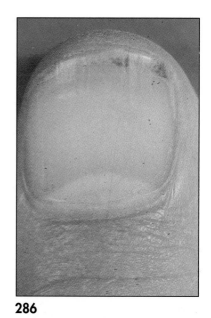

286

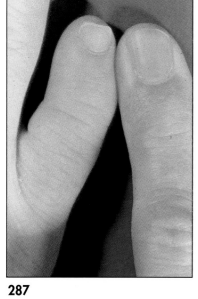

287

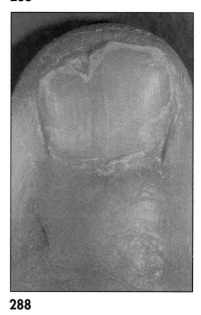

288

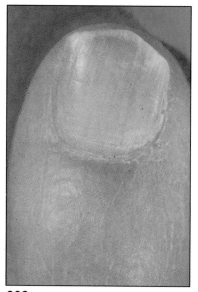

289

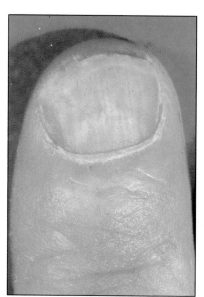

290

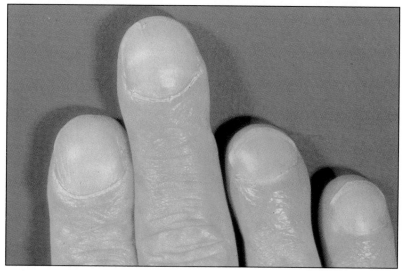

291

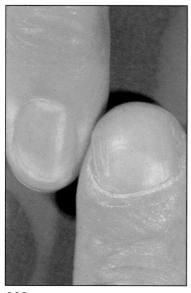

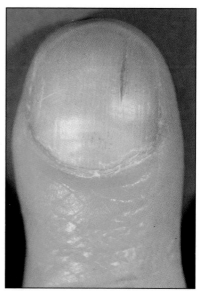

292

293

289 and 290   Elderly Down's. Nails from a long-surviving 64-year-old man with trisomy 21 (**289**). Thumbnail shows short, broad and convex nail with poorly developed lunula. (**290**) First finger, also short, broad nail—some thinning of nail near free edge.

291–293   Intellectual disability, trisomy 21, with Eisenmenger's syndrome and pulmonary stenosis. Note elongated middle finger and marked clubbing which has dominated nail development. (**291**) View of elongated finger. (**292**) Normal adult 1st finger from a person of the same age, showing enlargement of fingertip.(**293**) Drumstick clubbing and marked cyanosis; lunula unduly large and pale.

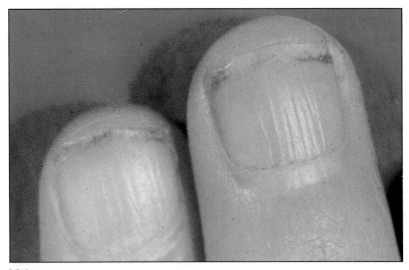

294

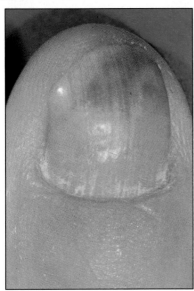

295

294 Normal length nails. Fingernails from Down's syndrome show abnormal longitudinal ridging and lack of manicure seen in association with mental disability.

295 Close-up of psoriatic nail-like appearance.

296 Monosomia 4. Totally absent lunula in a young woman with severe intellectual impairment, tapered fingers, lax ligaments and monosomia 4. Note appearance of "splinter" haemorrhages which are actually petechial dots.

297 Trisomy 7? Possible trisomy 7 with severe mental retardation and dysmorphia of skull. Some hypotoma, but marked incurving of 5th finger and narrow convex nail with no lunula.

298 Profound disability—trisomy 8. Minor changes in hands, incurving 5th finger and marked dysplasia of nails.

299 Monosomia 9. Monosomia 9 with severe psychosis and mental disability. Nails widened, with some lysis.

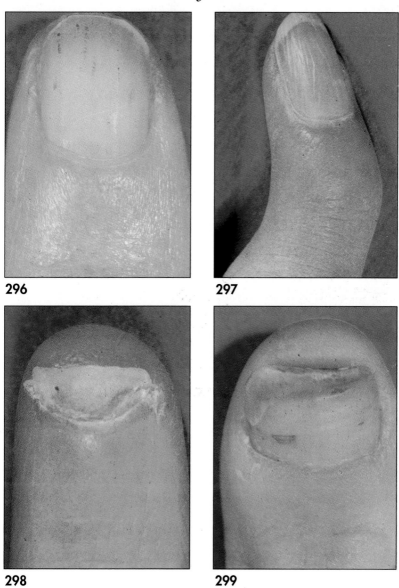

296

297

298

299

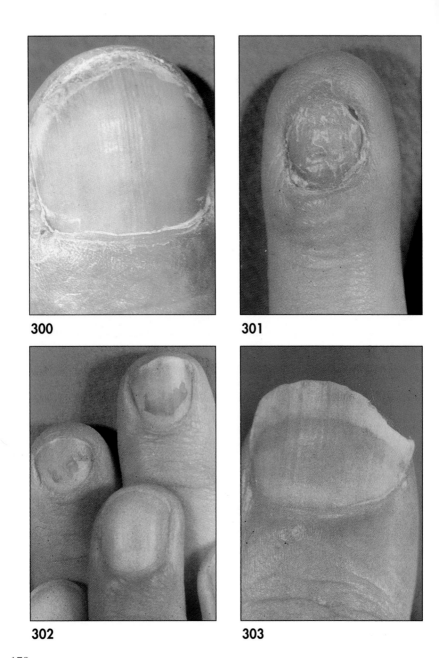

300

301

302

303

178

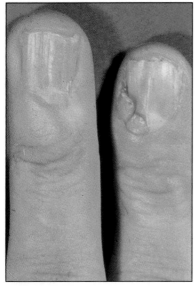

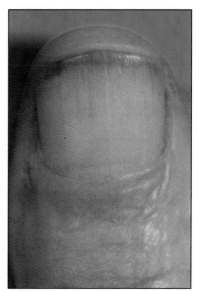

304   **305**

300   Quadrosomy X. Nails from middle-aged male with moderate retardation and double Klinefelter's syndrome. Patient shows quadrosomy X with mosaicism and incurving 5th finger. Thumbnails short, rounded and convex.

301   Gross nail dystrophy. Dyskeratosis congenita. Repeated shedding of nails since birth in a young, intellectually impaired woman.

302   Cri du chat sydrome. Note that nails are short and slightly convex, with longitudinal ridges unusual in a 20-year-old. Shown with normal nails of a female of the same age.

303   Wide "flared" nail. Microcephaly, profound mental retardation. Short, wide nails with no lunula and onycholysis. Chromosome status unknown.

304   Epiloia (tuberose sclerosis). Subungual fibromata seen in both middle and index fingers of the right hand in a woman mentally damaged from repeated fits.

305   Poor lunula. Microcephaly, mental disability and short nails with marked longitudinal ridging and poorly developed lunula. Monosomia 4?

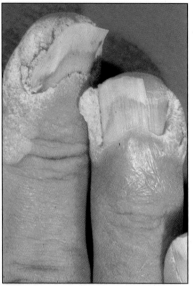

306

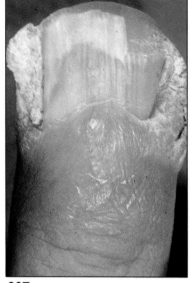

307

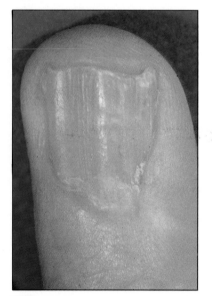

308

306 and 307 Gross dystrophy. Paraneoplastic acrokeratosis. Abnormalities of nail fold and secondarily of the nail. Normally appears in association with low-grade malignancy in respiratory or alimentary tract in men. Here seen in a mentally disabled patient with microcephaly (Bereau *et al.*, 1971).

308 Small pterygium. Young female with low IQ and tuberose sclerosis and fits. Middle fingernail shows pterygium secondary to very small early fibroma.

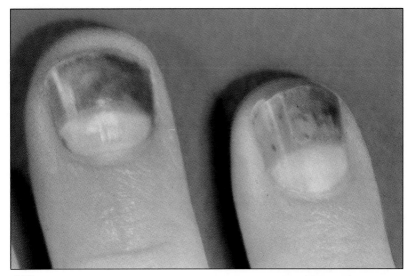

309

309 Aminoacidura. Intellectual disability, epilepsy and cystinuria with marked nail dystrophy. This young woman also had laxity of ligaments and tall stature.

310 Face and nail syndrome. Thumbnail dystrophy in 40-year-old, moderately disabled male with facial abnormalities. Chromosomes not yet studied.

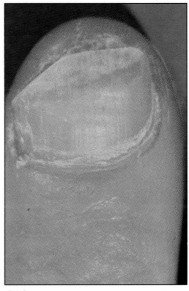

310

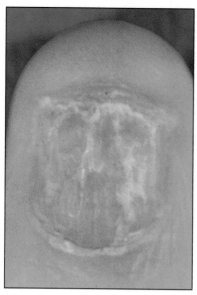

311

311 Dyskeratosis congenita. Also intellecually disabled with microcephaly.

312–314 Noack's or Pfeiffer's syndrome. Noack's syndrome with polysyndactyly and grossly abnormal nails. Trisomy 13?

312 (Noack's syndrome.) Convex micronychia in fused digits.

313 (Noack's syndrome.) Extreme micronychia of thumb.

314 (Noack's syndrome.) The "normal" nails show loss of lunula and convexity.

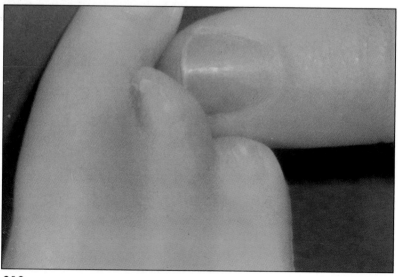

312

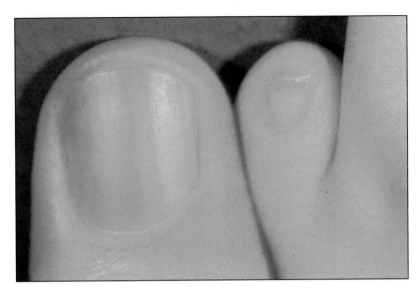

313

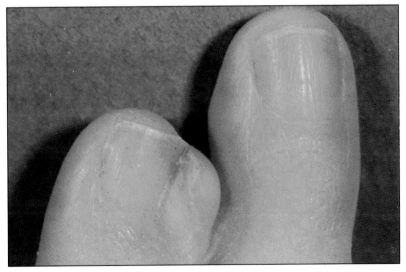

314

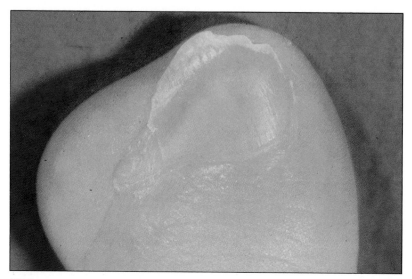

315

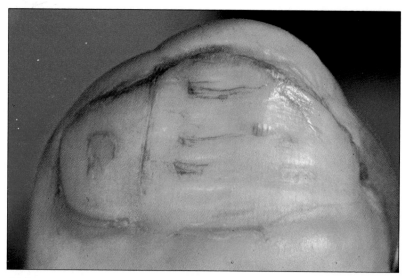

316

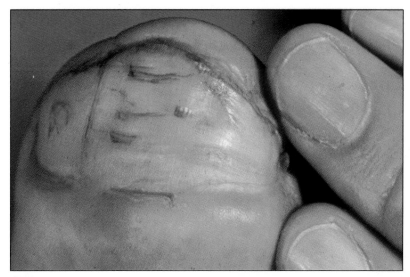

317

315 (Noack's syndrome.) Gross abnormality of thumb of right hand.

316 Apert's syndrome. Oxycephaly, mental impairment and hypertelorism with syndactyly. Note the fusion of 4 digits results in a single large nail. The thumb takes on a "flipper"-like role, convex and without lunula.

317 (Apert's syndrome.) Syndactyly of left hand (normal adult fingers alongside).

318 Close-up of thumb to show convexity and absence of lunula. Contrary to reports, there is no real atrophy of nail, but a fusion of all.

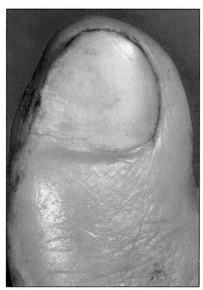

318

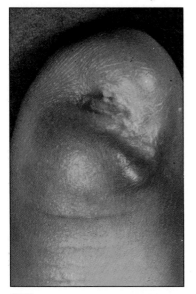

319

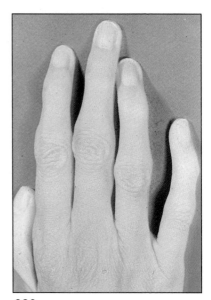

320

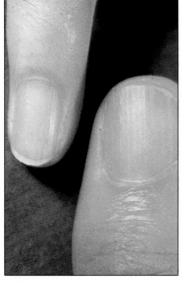

321

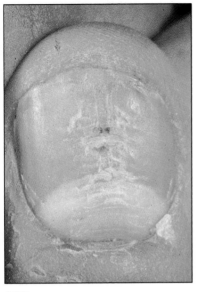
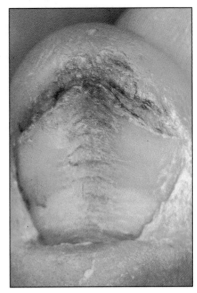

322   **323**

319   Amniotic nail syndrome. Nail of 5th finger absent since birth due to reduced amniotic fluid. All other nails normal.

320 and 321   Marked arachnodactyly. Intellectual impairment—arachnodactyly and homocysteinuria in an adult woman with long tapered fingers and nails. (**320**) Note incurving of 5th finger and length of digits. (**321**) Micronychia and elongation of nails in the 5th finger is clearly visible when compared to a normal nail.

322 and 323   Severe intellectual impairment from birth with central nail dystrophy. (**322**) Left thumbnail. (**323**) Right thumbnail resembles Leclercq canaliformis changes, but is almost certainly due to repetitive trauma.

References

1. Baran, R. in *The Nail*, Pierre, M. (ed), Churchill-Livingstone, London, 1981, pp. 20–24.
2. Boxley, J. D. Pachyonychia congenita and multiple epidermal haematomata. *British Journal of Dermatology*, 1971, **85**, 98.
3. Franzot, J., Kansky, A. & Kav'Ci'C, S. Pachyonychia congenita (Jadassohn–Lewandowsky syndrome). A review of 14 cases in Slovenia. *Dermatologica*, 1981, **162** (6), 462.
4. Gass, S. F., Guberman, R. M., D'Orazi, S. T. & Furci, T. J. Heritable nail diseases. *Clin–Podiatr–Med–Surg*, 1989, **6** (2), 339–45.
5. Gladen, B. C., Taylor, J. S., Wu, Y. C., Ragan, N. B., Rogan, W. J. & Hsu, C. C. Dermatological findings in children exposed transplacentally to heat-degraded polychlorinated biphenyls in Taiwan. *British Journal of Dermatology*, 1990, **122** (6), 799–808.
6. Goodman, R. M. & Cuppage, F. E. The nail patella syndrome. Clinical findings and ultrastructural observations in the kidney. *Archives of Internal Medicine*, 1967, **120**, 68.
7. Greenspan, D. S., Byers, M. G., Eddy, R. L., Cheng, W., Jani-Sait, S. & Shows, T. B. Human collagen gene COL5A1 maps to the q34. 2.q34.3 region of chromosome 9, near the locus for nail–patella syndrome. *Genomics*, 1992, **12** (4), 836–837.
8. Hazelrigg, D. E., Duncan, C. & Jarratt, M. Twenty nail dystrophy of childhood. *Archives of Dermatology*, 1977, **113,** 75.
9. Heimer, W. L., Brauner, G. & James, W. D. Dermatopathia pigmentosa reticularis: a report of a family demonstrating autosomal dominant inheritance. *Journal of the American Academy of Dermatology*, 1992, **26** (2Pt 2), 298–301.
10. Hodson, E. M., Kluckow, M. R. & O'Neill, P. Clinical quiz. Nail–patella syndrome (NPS) (hereditary osteo–onychodysplasia). *Journal of Pediatric Nephrology*, 1992, **6** (3), 314–16.
11. Nevin, N. C., Thomas, P. S., Calvert, J. & Reid, M. M. Deafness, onycho–osteodystrophy, mental retardation (DOOR) syndrome. *American Journal of Medical Genetics*, 1982, **13** (3), 325.
12. Ning, Y., Yongshan, Y., Pai, G. S. & Gross, A. J. Heterozygote detection through bleomycin-induced G2 chromatid breakage in dyskeratosis congenita families. *Cancer Genetics & Cytogenetics*, 1992, **60** (1), 31–4.
13. Noack's also Pfeiffer's syndrome, in *Mendelian Inheritance in Man*, McKusack, V.A. (ed.), 5th Edition, John Hopkins University Press, Baltimore, 1978, p. 8.
14. Pai, G. S., Morgan, S. & Whetsell, C. Etiologic heterogeneity in dyskeratosis congenita. *American Journal of Medical Genetics*, 1989, **32** (1), 63–66.
15. Parikh, A., Vaidya, V. U., Bharucha, B. A. & Kumta, N. B. Pachyonchia congenita *Journal of Postgraduate Medicine*, 1989, **35** (3), 189–90.
16. Patiroglu, T. & Hasanoglu, E. Anonychia associated with ectrodactyly syndrome: *Turkish Journal of Pediatrics*, 1989, **31** (93), 249–52.

17. Patrizi, A., Di Lernia, V. & Patrone, P. Palmoplantar keratoderma with sclero-dactyly (Huriez syndrome). *Journal of the American Academy of Dermatology,* 1992, **26** (**5** Pt 2), 855–7.

18. Pfeiffer, R. A. The oto–onycho–peroneal syndrome. A probably new genetic entity. *European Journal of Pediatrics,* 1982, **138**, 317.

19. Pinheiro, M. & Freire-Maia, N. Hair–nail dysplasia—a new pure autosomal dominant ectodermal dysplasia. *Journal of Clinical Genetics,* 1992, **41** (96), 296–8.

20. Reichel, M., Grix, A. C. .& Isseroff, R. R. Dyskeratosis congenita associated with elevated fetal haemoglobin, X-linked ocular albinism, and juvenile-onset diabetes mellitus. *Pediatric Dermatology,* 1992, **9** (2), 103–6.

21. Rider, M. A. Congenital palmar nail syndrome. *Journal of Hand Surgery,* 1992, **17** (3), 371–2.

22. Ronchese, F. The racket thumb nail. *Dermatologica,* 1973, **146**, 199.

23. Sharma, V. K., Sharma, R. & Kaur, S. Pachyonchia congenita with tuberous sclerosis. *Int. J. Dermatol.,* 1989, **28** (5), 332–333.

24. Sparrov, G. P., Samman, P. D. & Wells, R. S. Hyperpigmentation and hypo-hidrosis. *Clinical and Experimental Dermatology,* 1976, **1**, 127.

25. Stieglitz, J. B. & Centerwall, W. R. Paronychia congenita (Jadassohn–Lewandowsky syndrome): a seventeen-member, four-generation pedigree with unusual respiratory and dental involvement. *American Journal of Medical Genetics,* 1983, **14** (1), 21.

26. Takeda, Y., Itagaki, M. & Ishibashi, K. Hypoplastic–hypocalcified enamel of teeth and dysplastic nails: an undescribed ectodermal dysplasic syndrome. *Int. J. Oral Maxillofac. Surg.,* 1989, **18** (2), 73–5.

27. Tonoki, H., Kishino, T. & Niikaw, N. A new syndrome of dwarfism, brachy-dactyly, nail dysplasia, and mental retardation in sibs. *American Journal of Genetics,* 1990, **36** (1), 89–93.

28. Tosto, A., Fanti, P. A. & Varotti, C. Massive lymphomatous nail involvement in Sézary syndrome. *Dermatologica,* 1990, **181** (2), 162–164.

29. Tosti, A., Paoluzzi, P. & Baran, R. Doubled nail of the thumb. A rare form of polydactyly. *Dermatology,* 1992, **184** (3), 216–18.

30. Vuillaume, M., Daya-Grosjean, L., Vincens, P., Pennetier, J. L., Tarroux, P., Baret, A., Calvayrac, R., Taieb, A. & Sarasin, A. Striking differenced in cellular catalase activity between two DNA repair-deficient diseases: xeroderma pig-mentosum and trichothiodystrophy. *Carcinogenesis,* 1992, **13** (3), 321–8.

31. Zimmerman, P., Prior, J., McGuire, J., Harvey, J. Onychia of a macronychia in congenital aphalangia. *Journal of the American Podiatric Medical Association,* 1992, **82** (7), 380–1.

Chapter 13

Chromonychias or Coloured Nails

White nails or leukonychia are the most obvious and most helpful sign for an early medical diagnosis. Once one has excluded general medical conditions or skin conditions as the cause of white nails, then other coloured nails are likely to be due to common disorders—for example, drugs or fungus. In taking into consideration all of the reasons for coloured nails presenting to primary health workers, the most common causes are drugs (prescription), occupational ingestion of metals, and fungal or other infections.

The presentation of coloured nails demands a good history taking, and can be related to the increasing age of the patient—i.e. the transparency and thinness of the nail plate seen in many old people. The condition of the patient's blood is a factor in nail colour—i.e. anaemia results in pale or pink nail,s and reduced haemoglobin gives lilac or blue nails—as is the condition of the blood vessels—i.e. vasospasm and paleness (feel coolness of fingertips).

The main abnormalities in colour require an excellent light source, preferably sunlight. Changes in colour can be divided into three main groupings: those dependent upon whether the chromogenic agent is being applied from outside, as in certain occupations; those other dyschromias arising from within the nail bed or nail plate, which are usually classified as endogenous (of these, white nails or leukonychia are the most common and important); and the more general types. These categories are set out in Table 4.

TABLE 4. *A General Classification*

1. *White nails or leukonychias*

Nail plate
- Total leukonychia.
- Partial leukonychia
- Striated leukonychia.
- Congenital leukonychia.

Subungual leukonychia
- Terry's white nails.
- Muehrke's white bands.
- Uraemic "half-and-half" nails.
- Dermatology disorders, e.g. psoriatic white nails.

2. *Exogenous chromonychias*
- External applications, e.g., silver nitrate, gentian violet, etc.
- Cosmetics.
- Occupational, i.e., hairdressers and those working with
- French polish and varnish.
- Trauma..

3. *Endogenous dyschromias*

Toxic and therapeutic
- Poisons such as lead, silver, arsenic, etc.
- Drugs such as phenothiazines, anti-malarials, tetracyclines.
- Anti-mitotic drugs.
- Anti-fungal drugs.
- Drugs causing platelet changes and haemorrhages.

Systemic disorders, infections and nail bed pathologies
- Blood stream colours such as bilirubin and carotenaemia, etc.
- The yellow nail syndrome associated with lymphatic diseases.
- Pigmented nails associated with endocrine disorders.
- Melanonychia (pregnancy drugs , endrocrine diseases and malignant melanoma).
- Other cardiovascular, metabolic and congenital diseases such as Wilson's disease, polycythaemia, beri-beri, anaemia, other hypoalbuminaemias, etc.
- Infections. Examples would be the black and brown nails seen in onychomycoses, the green nails of *Pseudomonas*, yellow nails of *Scopulariopsis*, white nails of aspergillosus, etc.
- Lunulae changes.
- Red lunulae.
- Pigmented lunulae.
- Pigmented nail secondary to melamoma.

White Nails or Leukonychias

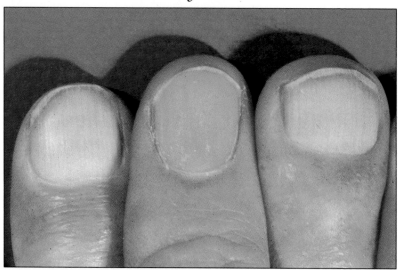

324

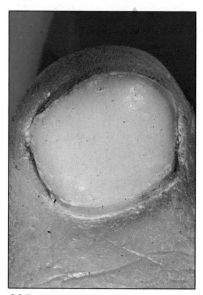

325

324 Leukonychia—tinge of cyanosis. Mentally disabled 60-year-old with mitral incompetence and congestive heart failure. Drug treatment has led to a mild dermatitis. Note bluish fingernails when compared with normal adult of same age. Nail with relative loss of lunula and bluish appearance of nail plate.

325 Leukonychia. Opaque white nails seen in a male in his 30s with alopecia totalis.

326 and 327 Chronic liver disease. Chronic persistent hepatitis (non-alcoholic) in post-menopausal woman. Note whiteness of all nails (serum albumen only 2.8g/l) and marked palmar erythema.

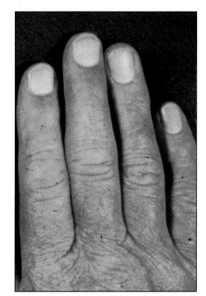

326

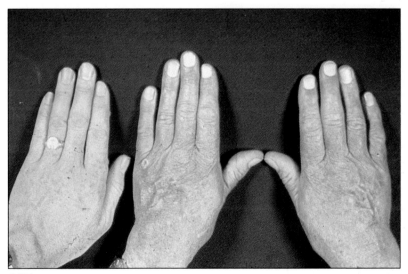

327

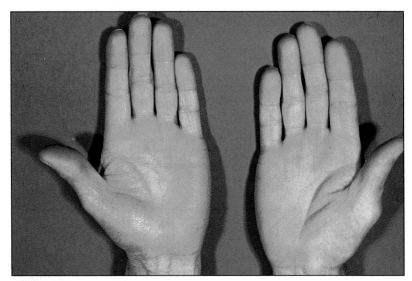

328

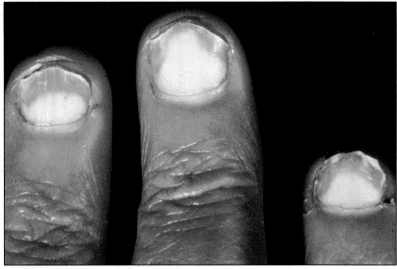

329

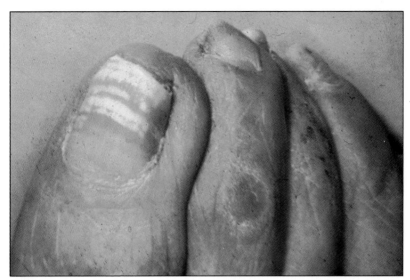

330

328   Palmar surface of nails shown in **327**.

329   Variable leukonychia. Hand of patient with marked renal failure and low serum albumen showing half and half nails.

330   Leukonychia striata in an elderly woman, probably due to repeated trauma to nail fold.

331   Striking half-and-half white nails in a woman with psoriasis.

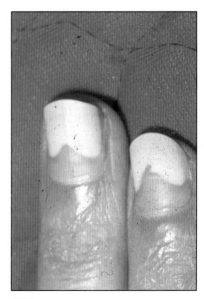

331

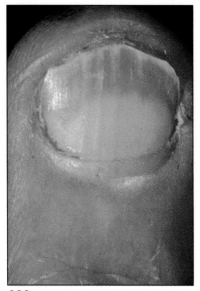

332

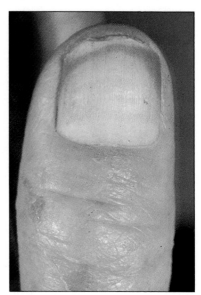

333

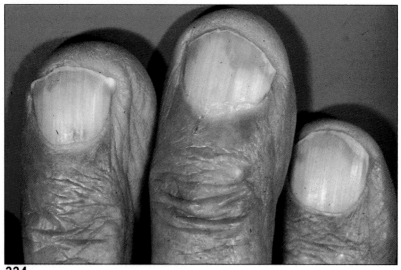

334

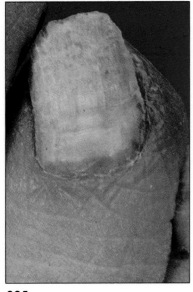

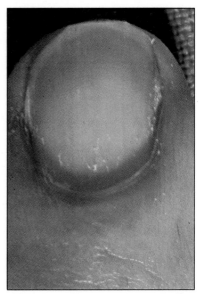

335 **336**

332 Half-and-half nail. A good example of Terry's half-and-half nails, this time due to renal failure.

333 Multiple changes with white nails. Coloured nail of a middle-aged male with chronic heart failure secondary to valvular disease. Cyanosis and slight jaundice are present, and the brown line under the free edge is secondary to nitrogen retention. The renal failure appears related to the low output state in this neglected patient. Note manicure.

334 Marked leukonychia. Severe total leukonychia in elderly patient with renal failure. Note small area of onycholysis and pigmented skin of organ failure.

335 Chromatodystrophy. Yellow-white chalky nails in a patient with Down's syndrome.

336 Unusual distal colouring. Terminal or distal nail discolouration in renal failure. The more usual nail signs are a thin dark brown line behind the yellow line or loss of lunula.

Yellow Nails

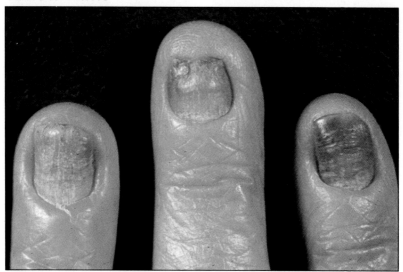

337

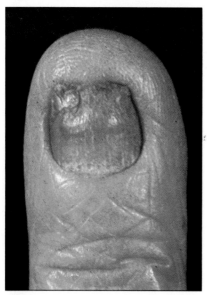

338

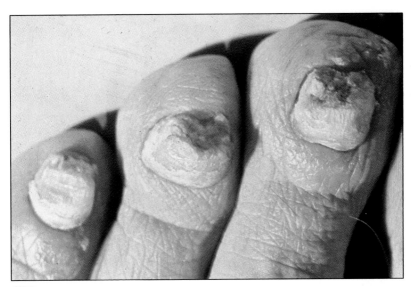

339

337 Yellow nails. Yellow nail syndrome seen in lymphatic abnormalities, especially thoracic and intestinal lymphangiectasia (Samman & White, 1964; Hiller *et al.*, 1972).

338 Yellow nail. Congenital abnormality of lymphatics with yellow nail dystrophy and secondary infection.

339 Yellow toenails. Yellow nail syndrome due to lymphatic hypoplasia in a 64-year-old farmer presenting with gross leg oedema and supposed diagnosis of congestive heart failure.

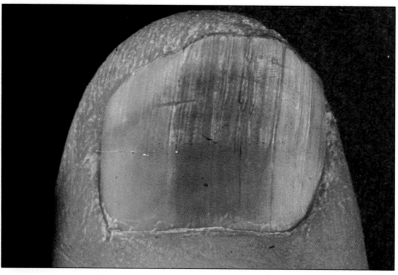

340

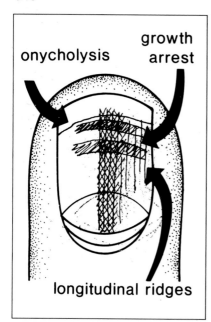

onycholysis

growth arrest

longitudinal ridges

340 Yellow-brown nails. Brown nails secondary to thyrotoxicosis in a middle-aged male of Caucasian decent. Note also marked distal onycholysis, growth arrest areas and prominent longitudinal nail ridges, also absent lunula.

341 Green nail syndrome. Pale green nail not in this case due to *Pseudomonas*. Exogenous pigment in damaged nail.

342 Green nail. Chronic *Pseudomonas* infection in toenail. Characteristic chronicity. May occur secondary to other skin diseases such as psoriasis (*see Chapter 15*).

343 Green–yellow nail. Green toenail seen in a man in his 30's who sustained a cricket ball injury to the end of the great toe as a teenager. No lymphatic abnormalities and no fungus in nail scrapings.

344 Acute *Pseudomonas* chromonychia.

Green Nails

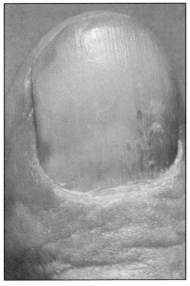

341

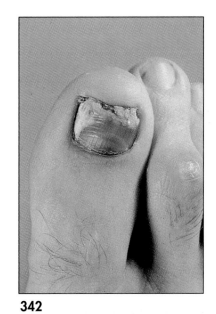

342

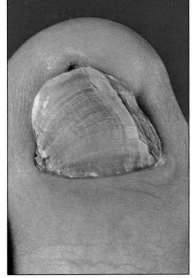

343

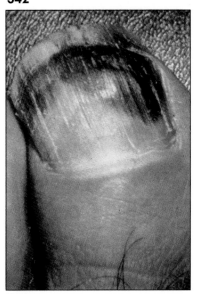

344

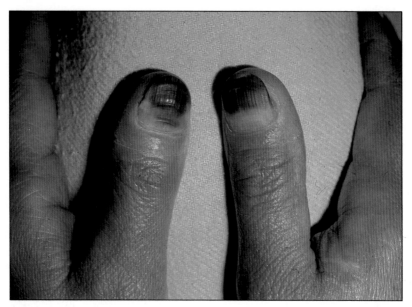

345

345 Both thumbs of **344**.

346 Thinning of nail—pink nail. A 60-year-old man with heart failure and very thin nails; thin nail plate presenting as pink nail. Note that lunula is just present.

347 Further "pink nail" due to thinning. Severe distal nail dystrophia in a 37-year-old man with "controlled" ulcerative colitis. Amyloid disease present on biopsy, etc. Amyloid nails as nail biopsy?

Pink, Mauve & Blue Nails

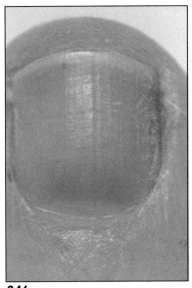

346

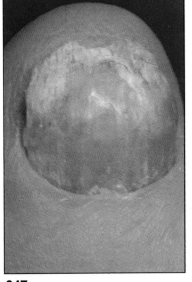

347

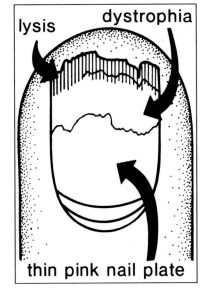

lysis dystrophia

thin pink nail plate

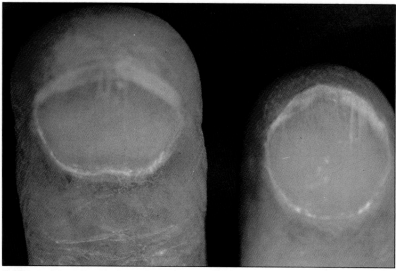

348

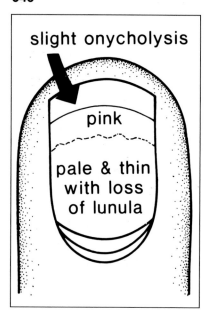

slight onycholysis

pink

pale & thin
with loss
of lunula

348 Pink nail syndrome. A 64-year-old widow with a marked nutritional disorder. Failure to eat adequate B and C vitamins as well as iron and protein results in pink nail syndrome. Nails flattened and thin, with loss of lunula and measured serum levels of iron, thiamine and vitamin C below lowest normal values.

349 Pink nail with striae. Loss of lunula in depressed 67-year-old widow. History of eating no protein but vegetables only. Serum albumen 3g/l. One small Beau's line and normal longitudinal striations.

350 Mauve nails. Mauve nails, combination cyanosis, whiteness and lack of lunular in a renal failure patient give this appearance. Note renal failure line under the free edge.

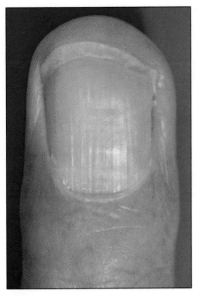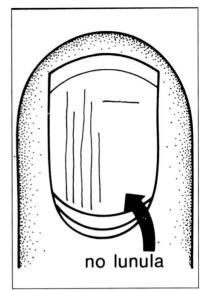

no lunula

349

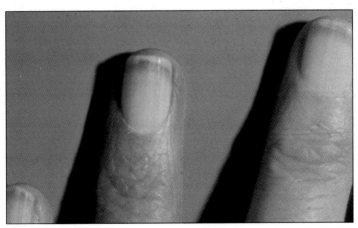

350

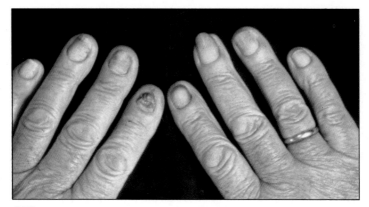

351

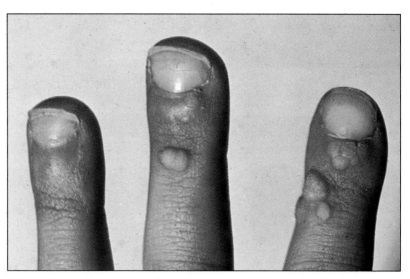

352

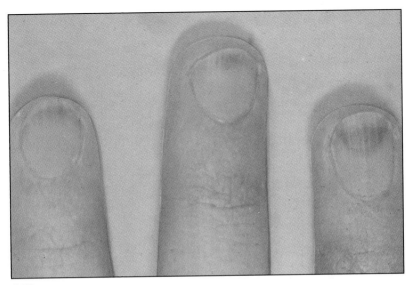

353

351 Dark mauve. Congestive heart failure which is chronic with cyanosis in a woman with Raynaud's disease of the hands. Note fungus of the nails.

352 Blue nails in child. Blue nail syndrome in a 10-year-old with colour change and hypertrophied terminal pulps since birth. Other congenital bone deformitities, but no lung or heart disease. Note also numerous viral warts.

353 Pale blue with pigment. Pigmentation on distal or leading edge of severe nails in a young woman. Probably due to drugs; possibly phenothiazines.

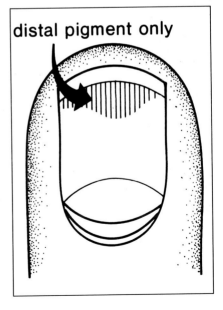

distal pigment only

Lilac & Brown Nails

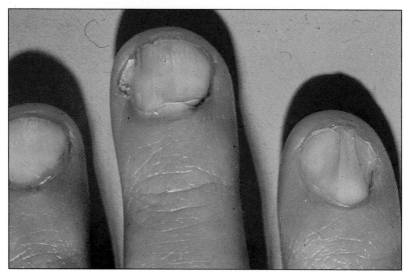

354

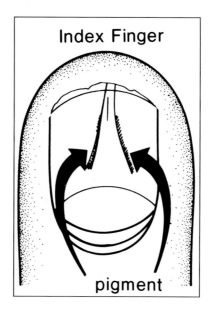

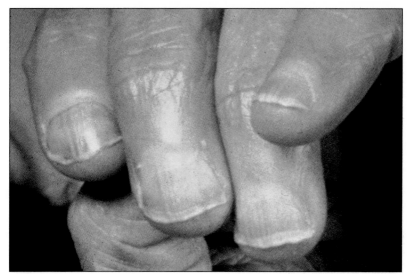

355

354 Pigment lines. Nail damage in a factory worker, due to fish packing with poor manicure of nails. Note also pigment lines in two nails.

355 Lilac nails. A 73-year-old woman with congenstive heart failure secondary to coronary heart disease, with poor appetite due to digoxin toxicity. Note "lilac" rather than blue colour. Also note poor care of nails.

356 Brown pigment in elderly chain smoker (stopped 7 weeks previously). Ridges related to age.

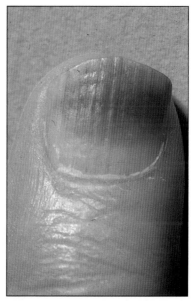

356

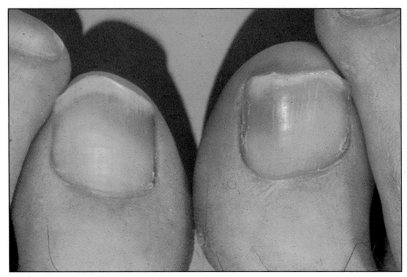

357

357 Kidney failure pigment. Brown lines of renal failure. Here seen in fingers, but better seen in toes. These brown lines spread further proximally as a discolouration.

358 General pigmentations. General pigmentations in thumbnails of a 70-year-old Chinese woman with 6 months of unexplained vomiting and weight loss. Chronic stress, no measurable nutritional abnormalities and no pathology found to account for condition. Note normal lunula and area of distal onycholysis.

359 Psoriatic pigmentation. Black nails due to psoriasis but not on treatment and no obvious skin lesions. Note also marked "pitting" of nails—resembling pottery "salt glaze".

360 Multifactorial pigmentation. Koilonychia (gross), some onycholysis and brown nails in a middle-aged, diabetic, Caucasian male with thyrotoxicosis and malnutrition.

210

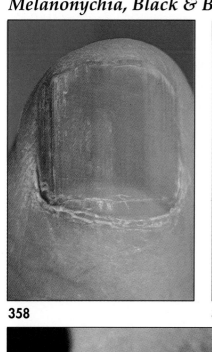

358

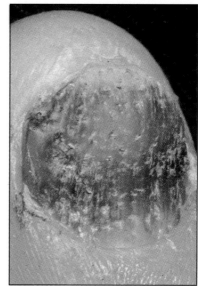

359

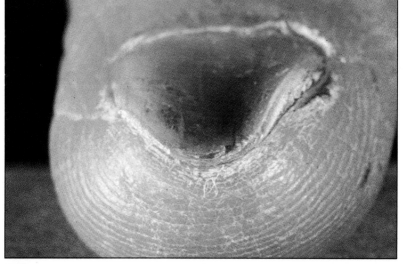

360

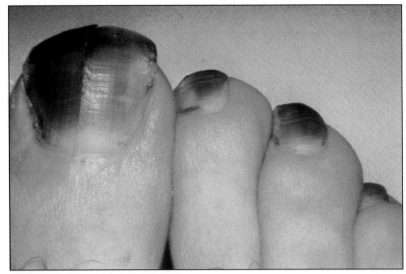

361

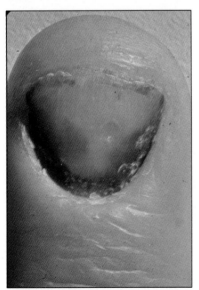

362

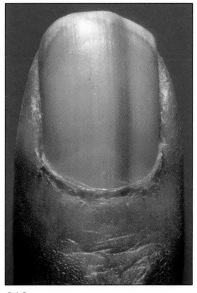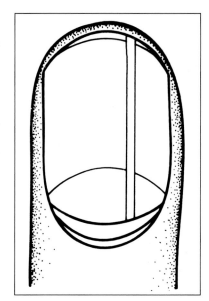

363

361 Pigment staining. Reddish-purple toenails due to staining with potassium permanganate (K_MNO_4).

362 Black arc pigment. Black proximal arc to nail plate, probably due to treatment of mild paronychia at nail base.

363 Brown line. Long, narrow, pigmented brown band in a male Caucasian. Addisonian with slow onset. A similar appearance is sometimes the result of a pigmented naevus at the base of the nail.

References

1. Anders, K. H. & Abele, D. C. Development of nail pigmentation during zidovudine therapy. *Journal of the American Academy of Dermatology,* 1989, **21** (4 pt 1), 792–3.
2. Daniel, C. R. Nail pigmentation abnormalities. *Dermatol. Clin.* 1985, **3**, 431–4.
3. Goldstein, G. D. & Dunn, M. I. Nailing down arsenic intoxication. *Chest,* 1989, **96** (93), 670–1.
4. Loveman, A. B. & Fliegelman, M. T. Discolouration of nails. *Archives of Dermatology,* 1955, **72**, 153.
5. Segal, B. M. Photosensitivity nail discolouration and onycholysis. *Archives of Internal Medicine,* 1963, **112**,165.
6. Weiss, E. & Sayegh-Carreno, R. PUVA-induced pigmented nails. *International Journal of Dermatology,* 1989, **28** (3), 188–9.
7. Wolf, R., Perluk, C. & Krakowski, A. Nail pigmentation resulting from selenium sulfide and copper. *In.t. J. Dermatol.,* 1989, **28** (8), 556–7.
8. Zhu, W. Y., Xia, M. Y., Haung, S. D. & Du, D. Hyperpigmentation of the nail from lead deposition. *Int. J. Dermatol.,* 1989, **28** (4), 273–5.

Green Nails

1. Chapel, T. A. & Adcock, M. Pseudomonas chromonychia. *Cutis,* 1981, **27**, 601.
2. Moore, M. & Marcus, M. D. Green nails: role of Candida (Syringospore monilia) and Pseudomonas aeruginosa. *Arch. Derm. Suph.* (Chicago), 1951, **64**, 49.

Melanonychias

1. Bendick, C., Rasokat, H. & Steigleder, G. K. Azidothymidine-induced hyperpigmentation of skin and nails. *Arch. Dermatol.,* 1989, **125** (9), 1285–6.
2. Fryer, J. M. & Werth, V. P. Pregnancy-associated hyperpigmentation: longitudinal melanonychia. *Journal of the American Academy of Dermatology.* 1992, **26** (**3** pt 2): 493–4.
3. Groark, S.P., Hood, A.F. & Nelson, K. Nail pigmentation associated with zidovudine. *J. Am. Acad. Dermatol.,* 1989, **21** (5 pt 1), 1032–3.
4. Hann, S. K., Hwang, S. Y. & Park, Y. K. Melanonychia induced by systemic photochemotherapy. *Photodermatol.,* 1989, **6** (2), 98–9.
5. Juhlin, L. & Baran, R. Longitudinal melanonychia after healing of lichen planus. *Acta Dermato-Venereologica* (Stockholm), 1989, **69** (4), 338–9.
6. Kamalam, A., Ajithadass, K., Sentamilselvi, G. & Thambiah, A. S. Paronychia and black discoloration of a thumb nail caused by Curvularia lunata. *Mycopathologia,* 1992, **118** (2), 83–4.
7. Kopt, A. W. & Waldo, E. Melanonychia striata. *Australian Journal of Dermatology,* 1980, **21** (2), 59.
8. Matsumoto, T., Matsuda, T., Padhye, A. A., Standard, P. G. & Ajello, L. Fungal melanonychia: ungual phaeohyphomycosis caused by Wangiella dermatitidis. *Clinical & Experimental Dermatology,* 1992, **17** (2), 83–6.
9. Saijo, S., Kato, T. & Tagami, H. Pigmented nail streak associated with Bowen's disease of the nail matrix. *Dermatologica,* 1990, **181** (2), 156–8.

10. Satanove, A. Pigmentation due to phenothiazines. *Journal of the American Medical Association,* 1965, **191,** 263.
11. Segal, B. M. Photosensitivity nail discolouration and onycholysis. *Archives of Internal Medicine,* 1963, **112,** 165.
12. Shelley, W. B., Rawnsley, H. M. & Pillbury, D. M. Post-irradiation melanonychia. *Archives of Dermatology,* 194, **90,** 174.
13. Stewart, W. K. & Raffle, E. J. Brown nail–bed arcs and chronic renal disease. *British Medical Journal,* 1972, **1,** 784.
14. Valero, A. & Sherf, K. Pigmented nails in Peutz–Jeghers syndrome. *American Journal of Gastroenterology,* 1965, **43,** 56.

Pigment Due to Melanomas

1. Kato, T., Usuba, Y., Takematsu, H., Kumasaka, N., Tanita, Y., Hashimoto, K., Tomita, Y. & Tagami, H. A rapidly growing pigmented nail streak resulting in diffuse melanosis of the nail. A possible sign of subungual melanoma *in situ. Cancer,* 1989, **64** (10), 2191–7.

Red Lunulae & Nails

1. Cohen, P. R. Red lunulae: case report and literature review. *Journal of the American Academy of Dermatology,* 1992, **26** (**2** Pt 2), 292–4.
2. Jorizzo, J. L., Gonzalez, E. B. & Daniels, J. C. Red lunulae in a patient with rheumatoid arthritis. *Journal of the American Academy of Dermatology*, 1983, **8** (5), 711.
3. Wilkerson, M. G. & Wilkin, J. K. Red lunulae revisited: a clinical and histopathologic examination. *J. Am. Acad. Dermatol.,* 1989, **20** (3), 453–7.

White Nails or Leukonychia

1. Ingegno, A. P. & Yatto, R. P. Hereditary white nails (leukonychia totalis), duodenal ulcer and gallstones. Genetic implications of a syndrome. *New York State Journal of Medicine,* 1982, **82** (13), 1797.
2. Jensen, O. White fingernails preceded by multiple transverse white bands. *Acta Dermato.Venereologica* (Stockh*),* 1981, **61** (3), 261.
3. Leyded, J. J. & Wood, M. G. The half-and-half nail of uremic onychodystrophy. *Archives of Dermatology,* 1972, **105,** 591.
4. Lindsay, P. G. The half-and-half nail. *Archives of Internal Medicine,* 1967, **119,** 583.
5. Morey, D. A. J. & Burke, J. O. Distinctive nail changes in advanced hepatic cirrhosis. *Gastroenterology,* 1955, **29,** 258.

Yellow Nail Syndrome & Yellow Lunulae

1. Buzio, C., De Martin, L. & De Palma, G. Pericarditis and the yellow nail syndrome (letter). *Annals of Internal Medicine.* 1992, **116** (10), 878–9.
2. Camilleri, A. E. Chronic sinusitis and the yellow nail syndrome. *J. Laryngol. Otol,* 1990, **104** (10), 811–3.
3. DeCoste, S. D., Imber, M. J. & Baden, H. P. Yellow nail syndrome. *J. Am. Acad. Dermatol.,* 1990, **22** (4), 608–11.

4. Govaert, P., Leroy, J. G., Pauwels, R., Vanhaesebrouck, P., De Praeter, C., Van Kets, H. & Goeteyn, M. Perinatal manifestations of maternal yellow nail syndrome. *Pediatrics,* 1992, **89** (**6** Pt 1), 1016–8.
5. Hendricks, A. A. Yellow lunulae with fluorescence after tetracycline therapy. *Archives of Dermatogy,* 1980, **116** (4), 438.
6. Miro, A. M., Vasudevan, V. & Shah, H. Ciliary motility in two patients with yellow nail syndrome and recurrent sinopulmonary infections. *Am. Rev. Respir. Dis.,* 1990, **142** (4), 890–1.
7. Lodge, J. P., Hunter, A. M. & Saunders, N. R. Yellow nail syndrome associated with empyema. *Clin. Exp. Dermatol.,* 1989, **14** (4), 328–9.
8. Tan, W. C. Dietary treatment of chylous ascites in yellow nail syndrome. *Gut,* 1989, **30** (11), 1622–3.

Chapter 14

Tumours & Pterygia

Warts and small periungual fibromata are the more common lesions presenting to the family doctor. A persistent, odd-looking or any pigmented lesion or tumour should **always** be referred on to a skin specialist for a second opinion, or biopsy, as it may be malignant. Examples of lesions and tumours most commonly seen, including rarer types, are set out in Table 5 (below).

Goldman (1992) and colleagues have drawn attention to the fact that periungual fibromas may be seen in association with tuberous sclerosis or Von Recklinghausen's disease. They may more likely arise *de novo*, but are "comparatively rare". Associated with the posterior nail fold and near the matrix cells, they have the potential for nail growth deformity, especially if "boxed in" by a shoe.

TABLE 5. *Commonly occurring tumours and lesions around and under the nails*

Commonly seen
- Warts
- Epidermoid cysts
- Fibromata
- Xanthoma
- Small myxomas
- Keloid formation

Uncommon but very important
- Melanotic & pigmented lesions [presenting late]
- Malignant melanoma
- Basal cell carcinoma / squamous cell carcinoma
- Sarcomata / metastases papillomas

Rare
- Multiple exostoses
- Enchondromata
- Tumours of neurogenic and angiomatous origin

Osteochondromas (Eliezri 1992) and subungal exostoses (Hoehn 1992) are very rare, and eventually present for excision. Ridge & Briggs (1992), in reviewing subungual melanomas, showed that 90% occurred under either the thumb or hallux nail, and consequently emphasised that delays in presentation or referral were usual.

Almost always, tumours around the nail plate presented to the family physician are subsequently referred on to a dermatologist with an interest in the nails. Warts and small periungual fibromata around the nail folds are the most common simple tumours, followed by mucous cysts and exostoses. Pigmented naevi, glomus tumours, keratocanthomas and epidermoid inclusions are all rare and need specialised advice and surgical removal.

The very rare nail bed cancers such as epitheliomata and malignant melanomas may be seen perhaps once in the practising lifetime of a general practitioner, usually in elderly patients. A malignant melanoma may present as a small pigmented area secondary to a small localised paronychia. It may also appear as a junctional naevus. The amelanotic melanomas under or near the nail, being difficult to diagnose, may present late (Ridge & Briggs 1992).

Pterygia

Most pterygia arise from small, penetrating injuries or disorders at the proximal end of the nail bed, deep enough to injure the matrix in a localised area. A prime example would be the small fibromata seen in epiloia, where pterygia are commonly seen in association with the many small nail fold fibromata. The term **dorsal pterygium** is often used where the nail fold grows down over the nail plate and lunula, and is almost always associated with skin diseases or damage to the terminal digit.

The so-called true or **ventral pterygia** are again sometimes associated with trauma, but if not related to Raynaud's or systemic sclerosis are usually due to inherited (familial) or congenital configuration of the distal groove. These are also called pterygium inversum unguis.

As Shukla and Hughes have stated:

"Benign subungual naevi are rare in Europeans,
all subungual naevi or pigments should be regarded as malignant until
proven otherwise."

364 Cyst of finger. A mucous or mucoid cyst of finger. Thought of as arising from the nail fold, but actually from collagenous degeneration of extensor tendon.
365 Tumours and cysts. Mucous cyst over dorsum of the finger arising from degeneration of tendon.
366 Cyst with nail changes. Mucoid cyst at base of nail bed with associated distal changes in the nail.

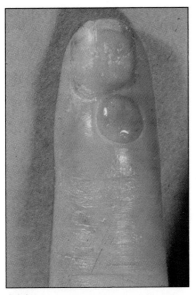

364

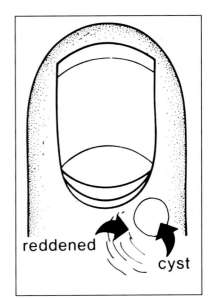

reddened

cyst

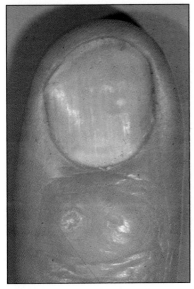

365

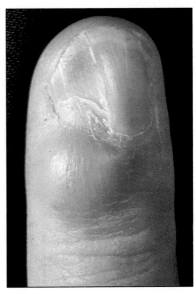

366

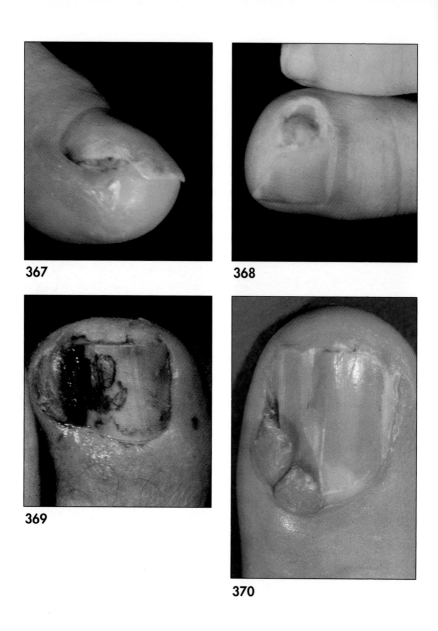

367

368

369

370

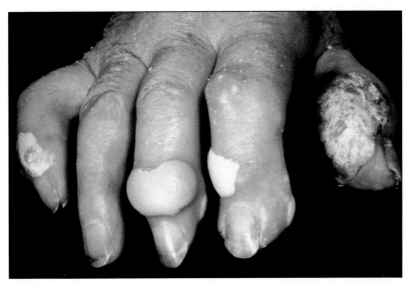

371

367 Subungual fibroma. Nail excised away above a subungual fibroma.
368 Subungual exotosis of great toe.
369 Nail bed tumour. Small mucoid tumour of great toenail bed (non-malignant).
370 Two subungual fibromata. Watch for other lesions, as sometimes seen with epiloia and calcified cerebral vessels.
371 Pseudo tumours. Nails and hands with chronic topaceous gout (extreme example).

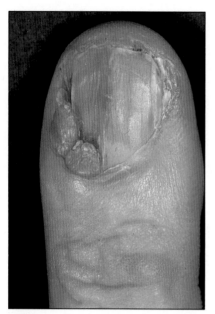

372

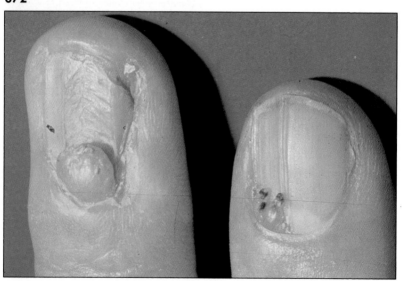

373

222

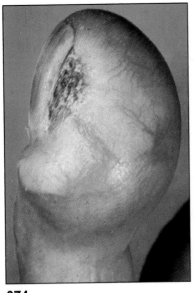

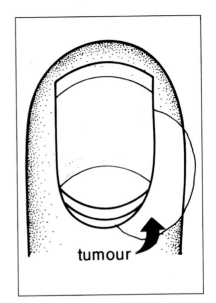

374

372 A double fibroma pushing up laterally from matrix cells.
373 Fibromata in two nails proximally with damage to distal part of nail plate.
374 Malignant tumour. Periungual malignant fibroma in a smoking pensioner. Note also "beaking" of the nail.
375 Sarcoma of the nail bed.

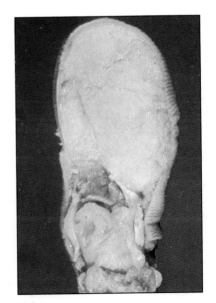

375

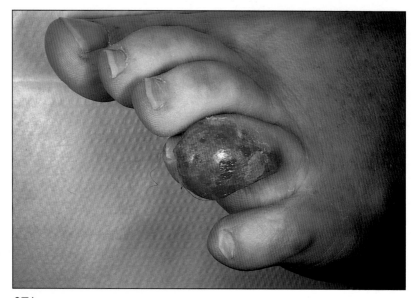

376

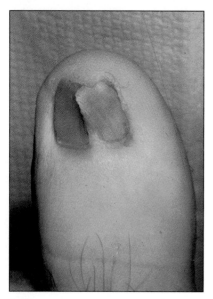

376 Advanced melanoma growing rapidly, having been neglected for a year because it started as an amelanotic melanoma at proximal base of nail (patient died 12 months later from secondaries).

377 Small pterygium (= prow of ship). Early pterygium on one nail only. No obvious cause, such as lichen planus, was found.

378 A median dystrophy presenting as bilateral pterygia.

377

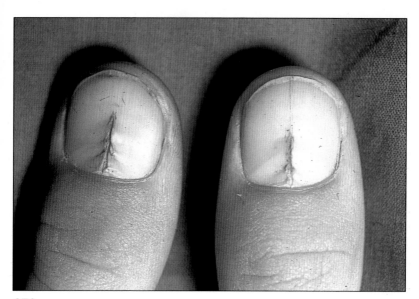

378

References

1. Baran, R. & Kint, A. Onychomatrixoma. Filamentous tufted tumour in the matrix of a funnel-shaped nail, a new entity (report of three cases). *British Journal of Dermatology,* 1992, **126** (5), 510–5.

2. Chin, F. E. & McCarthy, D. J. The cytological and biochemical implications of periungual fibroma. *Journal of Foot Surgery,* 1992, **31** (5), 486–97.

3. Eliezri, Y. D. & Taylor, S. C. Subungual osteochondroma. Diagnosis and management. *Journal of Dermatologic Surgery & Oncology,* 1992, **18** (8),753–8.

4. Evison, G. Subungual exostosis. *British Journal of Radiology,* 1966, **39**, 451.

5. Fanti, P. A. & Tosti, A. Subungual epidermoid inclusion, report of 8 cases. *Dermatologica,* 1989, **178** (4), 209–12.

6. Goldman, E. P., Boike, A. M. & Snyder, A. J. An unusual presentation of a periungual fibroma. *Journal of the American Podiatric Medical Association,* 1992, **82** (4), 215–7.

7. Gordon, M. & Palusci, V. J. Human papilloma virus type 16 periungual carcinoma. *JAMA,* 1989, 22–9; **262** (24), 3407–8.
8. Harvey, K. M. Pigmented naevus of nail. *Lancet,* 1960, **ii,** 848.
9. Hoehn, J. G. & Coletta, C. Subungual exostosis of the fingers. *Journal of Hand Surgery* (St Louis). 1992, **17** (3), 468–71.
10. Kaminsky, C. A., de Daminsky, A. R. & Shaw, M., Formentini, E. & Albulafia, J. Squamous cell carcinoma of the nail bed. *Dermatologica,* 1978, **157** (1), 48.
11. Leppard, B., Sanderson, K. V. & Behan, F. Subungual malignant melanoma, difficulty in diagnosis. *British Medical Journal,* 1974, **1,** 310.
12. Lewing, K. Subungual epidermoid inclusions. *British Journal of Dermatology,* 1969, **81,** 671.
13. Moy, R. L., Eliezri, Y. D., Nuovo, G. J., Zitelli, J. A., Bennett, R. G. & Silverstein, S. Human papillomavirus type 16 DNA in periungual squamous cell carcinomas. *JAMA,* **261** (18), 2669–73.
14. Ridge, H. S. & Briggs, J. C. Subungual melanoma, a clinico-pathological study of 24 cases. *British Journal of Plastic Surgery,* 1992, **45** (4), 275–8.
15. Saida, T. & Ohshima, Y. Clinical and histopathologic characteristics of early lesions of subungual malignant melanoma. *Cancer,* 1989, **63** (3), 556–60.
16. Salasche, S. J. & Orengo, I. F. Tumours of the nail unit. *Journal of Dermatologic Surgery & Oncology,* 1992, **18** (8), 691–700.
17. Shukla, V. K. & Hughes, L. E. How common are benign subungual naevi? *European Journal of Surgical Oncology,* 1992, **18** (3), 249–50.
18. Ward, P. E. & McCarthy, D. J. Periungual fibroma. *Cutis,* 1990, **46** (2), 118–24.

Chapter 15
Toenails

This section on toenails has been enlarged and expanded in response to many requests from podiatrists and chiropodists. Although toenails reflect general disorders in the same way as fingernails, there is a slower growth along the length of the nail plate. As the older age groups in all western societies become more numerous and important, long-term habits, and often inappropriate footwear, may show up to one year's changes in health status in the toenails.

Gravitational turbulence occurs increasingly down the whole length of the arterial tree. This arterial tree originally evolved 300 million years ago, with low pressure waves from a heart which was closer to the ground and short arteries to all four limbs. With the assumption of an upright posture and the need to pump blood to an enlarging and very high brain, the pressures are necessarily higher, and thus produce huge gravitational forces in the lower limb arteries. These forces also create turbulence, and so sludging or atheromatous plaques at the aortic bifurcation and in the narrower segments of the femoral or popliteal arteries.

Thus, evidence of reduced blood supply—and the assumption of more proximal atheromatous narrowing—is seen frequently in the toenails of the elderly western person, but seldom in the fingernails.

Deductions made from observations of the abnormal appearances of toenails have become increasingly important in many medical disorders. Such abnormalities are widely seen in ischaemia of the legs, stroke and heart attack patients, work and occupational groups and above all, in people with diabetes mellitus.

All of the sections which follow decsribe and illustrate changes seen commonly in people presenting to general internal medicine services with other disorders. Many of these examples are now used in tutorial classes at the New Zealand School of Podiatry.

Onychomycoses and ingrowing nails provide many referrals in the younger and middle-aged groups, as do peripheral vascular disease and onychogryphosis in the elderly. Above all, toenails, with their transverse ridging, rounding and frequent mycotic infections, reflect the effect of footwear. Although inadequately designed or unsuitable shoes and boots account for many of the changes seen in general practice or primary care examinations, rarely is further evidence from a visual inspection and feeling of the skin and an observation of the arteries sought, or advice from any deductions given.

Fungal Infections — Toenail

In the toes, one or occasionally more of the nails are usually involved, with a gradually developing, chalky opacity of the nail plate. The most common infections in the toes are *Trichophyton rubrum* and *Trichophyton interdigitale*. Other moulds are yeasts and may be grown in about half the cases where fungus infection is suspected from appearances in the toenails. The frequency of different types of infections is clearly related to the epidemiology of fungi, yeasts and moulds in that particular geographical area. Temperature and humidity are also critical factors. (See Chapter 5 for a discussion of onychomycoses.)

Aspergillus, Cephalosporium and *Scopulariopsis brevicaulis* may also be found in the toenails. The latter is usually confined to one great toe, giving a characteristic chalky, yellow appearance. As with this latter group of moulds, some sort of earlier damage to the nail or nail folds is needed for secondary fungal invasion to occur, but this can be water or persistent sweat damage.

Lastly, it is seldom recognised that occupational or footwear markings on the great toenails provide a unique indicator of differential growth—if this is too slow in one or both of the nails, it will signify proximal narrowing and reduced blood flow, especially if accompanied by signs of malnourishment such as flaking, scaling, thinness or shininess of the skin or widespread fungal infections in several nails.

Normal Variations

Each individual ethnic group or culture will show specific transverse ridges associated with the footwear of the group. In third-world countries, a wide variety of traumatic changes are seen in a variety of occupations where footwear may be uncommon or inadequate. Most of the changes seen in this and in the next section are those presenting to general medical service in teaching hospitals in New Zealand and Australia.

379 Normal. Healthy great toenail of a young female.

380 Normal—some transverse lines. Normal great toenail of woman given to wearing tights, who habitually wears open-toed sandals.

381 Normal. Great toenail from normal young female given to wearing tight "court" shoes.

382 Normal variations. Great toenail from normal young female. Note small area of distal onycholysis and some "ingrowing area on right margin".

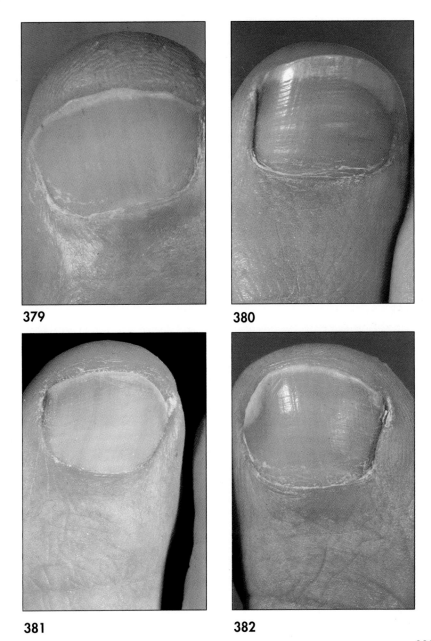

379

380

381

382

229

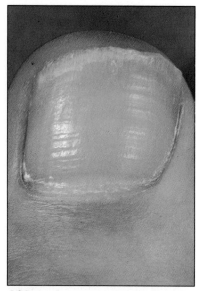

383

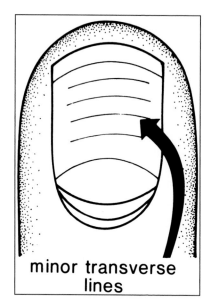

minor transverse
lines

383 Normal great toenail (of a receptionist). Transverse ridges due to customary use of tight high heels.
384 Great toenail of healthy male clerk (38 yrs)—eponychium growing over lateral grove, allowing early infection.

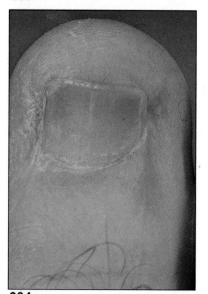

384

Minor & Congenital Changes

385 Congenital onychodysplasia syndrome. Additional nails usually in fingers, but in this teenage, intellectually disabled woman, the fingers were normal—one digit only.

386 Bifid digit and fused hifid nail in the hallux of a middle-aged Afro-American.

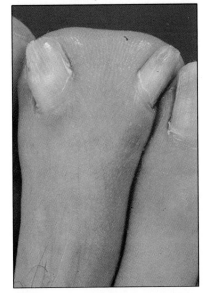

385

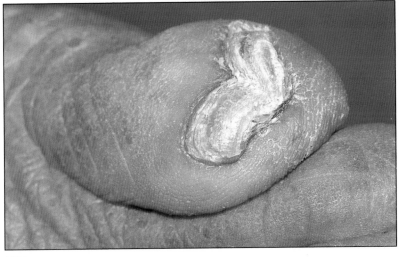

386

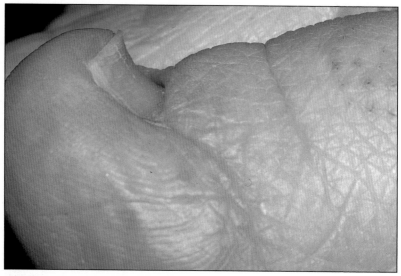

387

387 Great toenail of an achodroplastic dwarf, showing brachyonychia.
388 Mild trauma—blow from a digging spade.
389 Anchor dropped on right hallux of holidaying elderly physician 6 months previously.
390 Stumbling injury with small haematoma. Note opacity of nail and skin changes in a Pacific Island cargo worker.

Trauma of Toenails

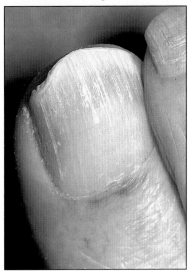

388

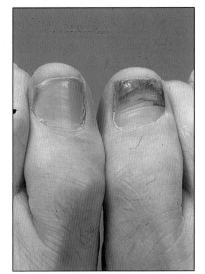

389

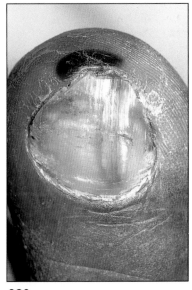

390

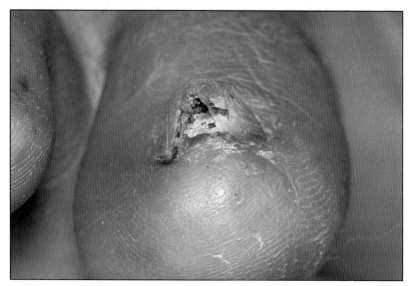

391

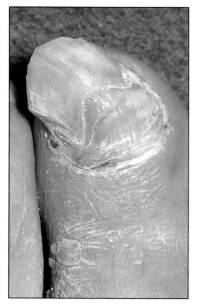

392

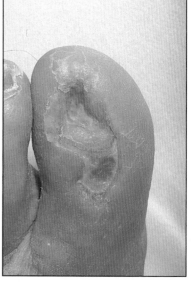

393

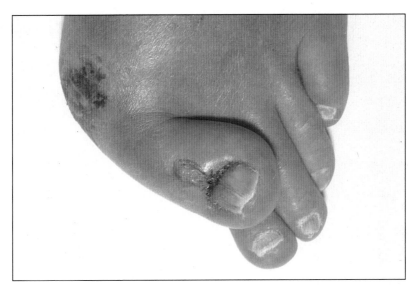

394

391 Central nail bed injury in a Maori patient.
392 Curved nail in a diabetic patient, the result of a previous injury.
393 Avulsion injury to nail bed, now healing cleanly.
394 Footwear injury in an alcoholic middle-aged barman with peripheral neuropathy.

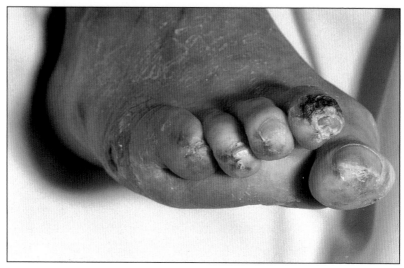

395

395 Footwear trauma in elderly woman with diabetes mellitus, experiencing loss of sensation.
396 Avulsed nail due to lawnmower injury.
397 Severe rotary mower ("Flymo") injury in barefoot gardener.

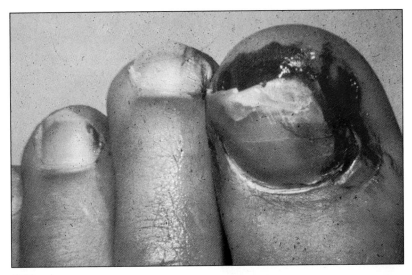

396

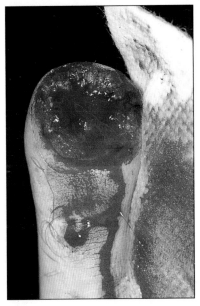

397

Fungus & Other Infections

Although some texts distinguish between bacterial and fungal infections, there remains much debate about the role of water content from immersion or sweat in allowing the breaking down of skin integrity. Nutritional factors are now regarded as important, and reactions to systemic drugs, as well as reduction in blood flow, willproduce changes in local immunity. Local "saprophytic" or skin-dwelling staphylococci may predate either bacterial infections by such organisms as *Candida*, *Coliforms* or *Pseudomonas*. Various dermatophytic fungal infections thus may be either primary or follow the above bacterial infections.

In all cases where chronic paronychia or widespread mycoses occur in the toenails, ischaemia, diabetes mellitus or occupational factors MUST be excluded.

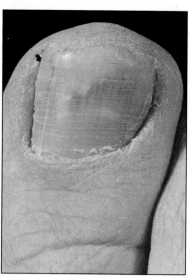

398

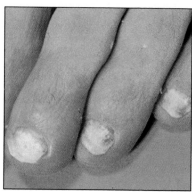

399

398 Fungus. Onychomycosis of great toe (*Trichophyton*) showing lysis and thickening.
399 Fungus (*Scopulariopsis*) in several toenails of a young man working in gumboots, confirmed by scrapings.
400 Several nails of a Samoan labourer infected with *Trichophyta*.
401 Simple nail fungus infection in a healthy squash player.
402 Mycotic infection on lateral edge of hallux—note drug-induced bleeding.

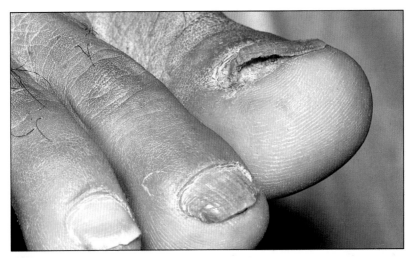

400

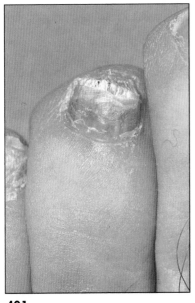

401

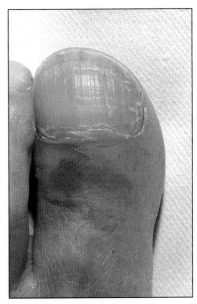

402

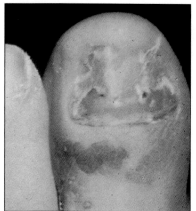

403

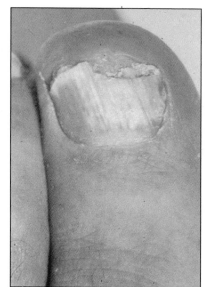

404

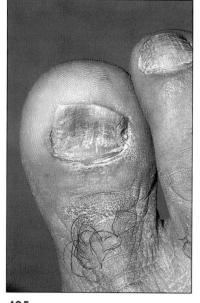

405

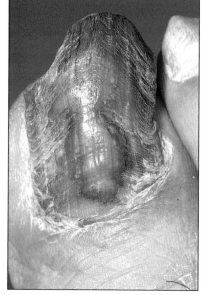

406

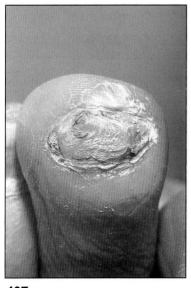

407

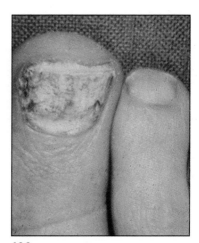

408

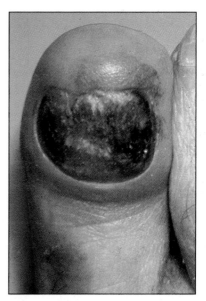

409

403 Infection. Excision of nail secondary to gross staphylococcal infection.

404 Great toe tinea. Onycho-mycosis or fungal infection of great toenail, giving rise to dystrophy.

405 "Black nail" syndrome in a Pacific Islander (fisherman) with chronic fungus in both toes.

406 Lifelong infection under toenail plate of an Afro-American driver.

407 Dairy worker in gumboots—trauma and chronic mycoses.

408 Onychomycosis with lifting and loss of toenails.

409 Secondary paronychia. Acute paronychia in great toenail subsequent to trimming of an onychogryphosis.

HIV Infections

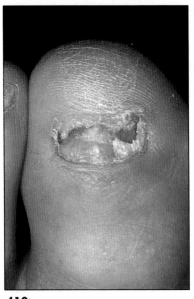

410

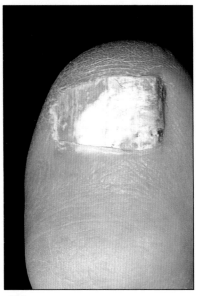

411

410 Recently admitted AIDS patient with neurologic syndrome in the left great toe.

411 Great toe of HIV-positive patient who experienced a reduced immunity over the previous few years—reduced immunity. No fungal growth.

412 Ischaemia. Great toenail of a man in his 60's with one leg amputated for vascular disease and second leg endangered. Note colour of skin which also has a 'waxy' appearance.

413 Proven (angiographic) severe atheroma with thin brittle nails. Some pigmentation and ridges in 70-year-old male ex-smoker.

414 Ischaemia rather than tinea. Nail dystrophy due to ischaemia of foot. Male, 68, long-term smoker with no run-off in angiogram. Note reddening and scaliness of skin.

415 Ischaemia. A 71-year-old man with heavy smoking history complaining of cold feet and poor eyesight (early cataract). Attempted home treatment of "ingrowing" toenail resulting in staphylococcal infection and necrosis in sulkus.

Ischaemic & Nutritional

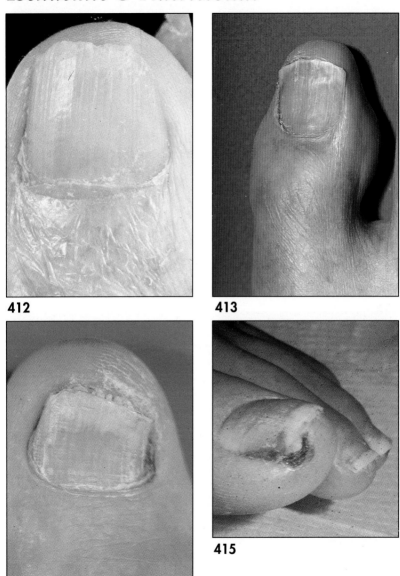

412

413

414

415

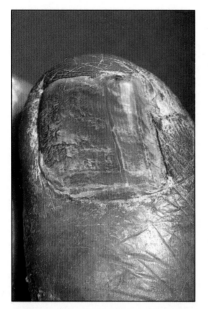

416

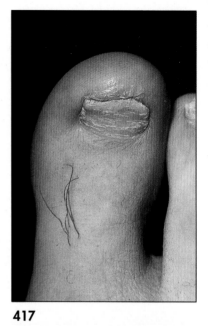

417

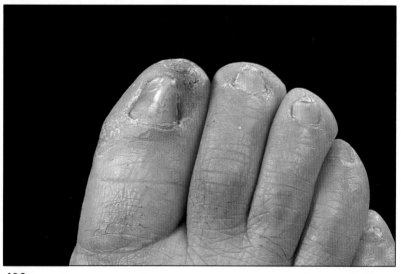

418

Medical Disorders

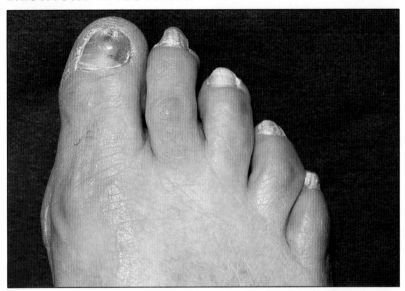

419

416 An 80-year-old ex-farmer with severe claudication in leg. Gross changes in skin and nail where mycotic infection is also present.

417 Ischaemic changes (colour change) and thin skin in a 50-year-old lifelong diabetic woman with absent femoral pulses.

418 Chronic, unremitting mycosis led to arterial studies (marked atheroma found) in a 60-year-old bank manager.

419 Foot of a 46-year-old woman with long-standing diabetes and chronic mycoses.

420 Managing a difficult paronychia in a diabetic man.

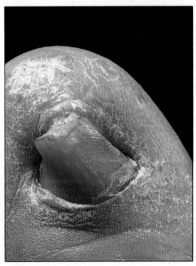

420

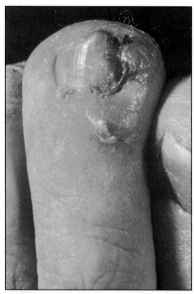

421 Unsuspected diabetes. Toe infection with nail damage secondary to long-standing but undiagnosed and untreated diabetes mellitus.

422 So-called "dry gangrene" in long-standing diabetes, with mild changes in hallux.

423 Most nails are dystrophic in long-standing diabetes with years of hyperglycaemia.

424 Diabetes of 40 years' duration, peripheral neuropathy with self- or auto-amputation of 2nd digit and marked ischaemic skin changes.

421

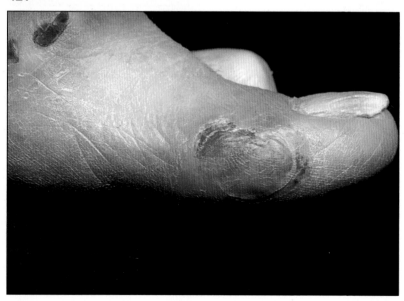

422

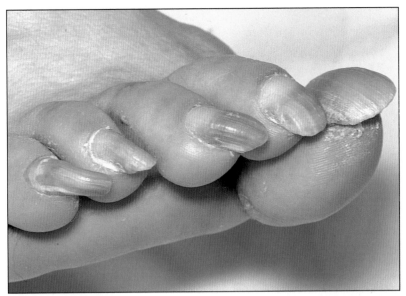

423

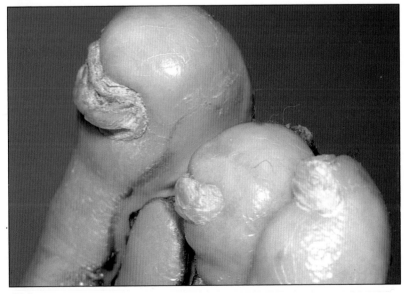

424

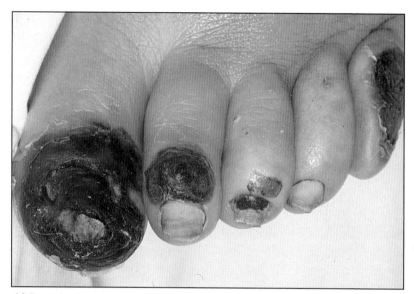

425

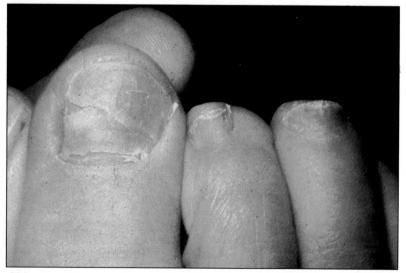

426

248

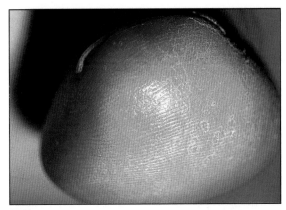

427

425 Gangrene in a 62-year-old neglected man with diabetes and peripheral neuropathy. Also, posible thiamin deficiency due to alcohol.
426 Raynaud's. "Shredding" of great toe of an elderly patient with Raynaud's disease.
427 End of nail and hallux in a man with disseminated lupus erythematosus.
428 Vasculitis in a young man with polyarteritis found on biopsy—drug related?
429 Lupus response in an elderly Afro-American man.

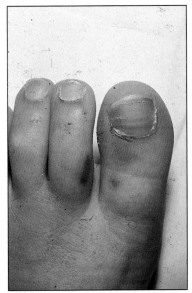

428

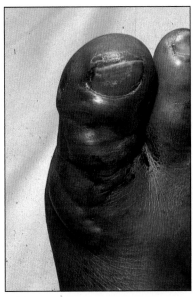

429

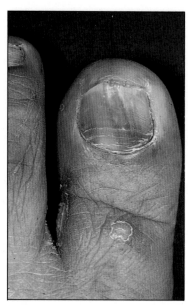

430 Toenail of 43-year-old Maori woman with Burkitts' lymphoma found during chemotherapy.

431 Severe unremitting Cushing's syndrome (persistently high cortisols and fungal infection).

432 Renal failure toenail in young male. Shows pigment and some thickening.

433 Clubbing of toes. Lateral view of marked clubbing in great toenails. Note lattice work of longitudinal ridges and some transverse lines.

434 Drug-induced purpura in a middle-aged male.

430

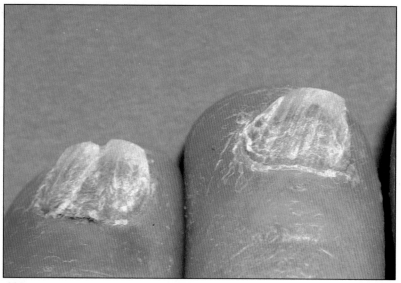

431

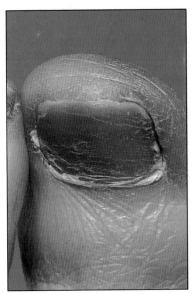

432

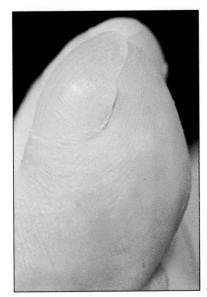

433

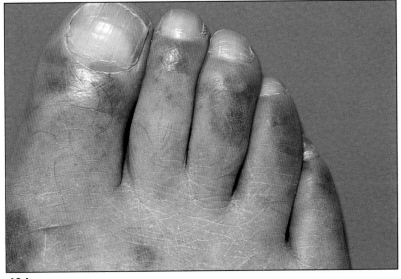

434

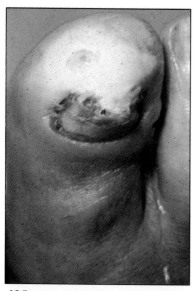

435

435 Peripheral neuropathy. Ulceration of tip of great toe secondary to peripheral neuropathy.
436 Pancreatic disease. Changes in great toe resulting from cystic fibrosis. No tinea found and no other skin lesions. Mechanism unknown.
437 Clubbing in toenail of young woman with bronchiectasis—note suggestion of splinter.

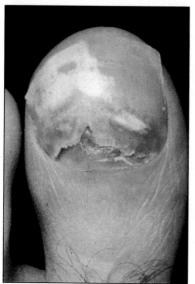

436

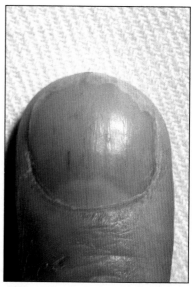

437

Coloured Toenails

438 "Greenness" due to trauma. Trauma to great toenail (weight dropped on toe) led to subungual haematoma.

439 Yellow nail syndrome: toenail involvement. Yellow nail syndrome in a man in his 60s who presented with hydrothorax and some swelling in the leg. This suggests lymphatic abnormalities in leg as well as in abdominal site.

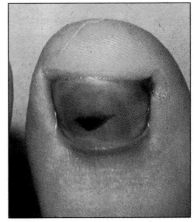

438

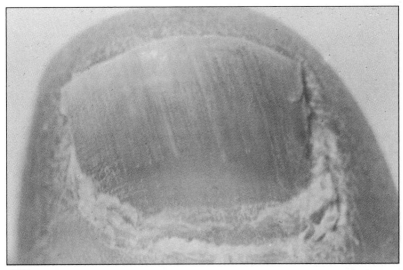

439

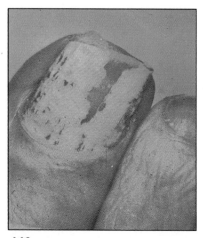

440

440 Chronic fungus. Chronic fungal infection leading to secondary staphlococcal paronychia and nail dystrophia in a diabetic patient with four times normal blood sugar level.

441 Mild yellow nail syndrome. Mild appearances of yellow nail syndrome in the toenails of a 56-year-old man with life-time history of congenital lymphatic abnormalities in the legs.

442 Red nail from fungicidal stain in a young woman.

443 Black toenails with thickened hallux nails, suggesting fungus—cause unknown.

444 Secondary paronychia. Acute paronychia in great toenail subsequent to trimming of an onychogryphosis.

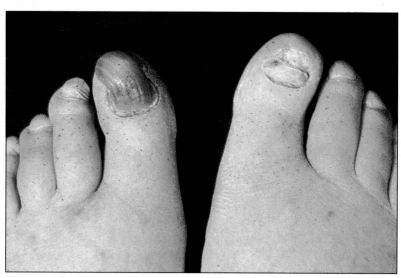

441

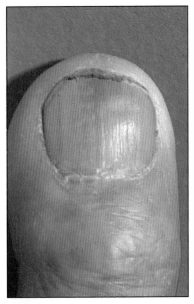

442

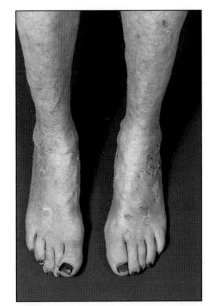

443

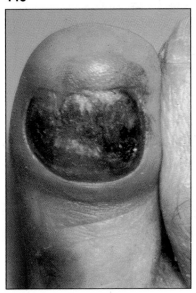

444

Other Skin & Toenail Disorders

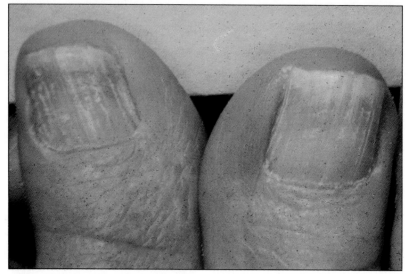

445

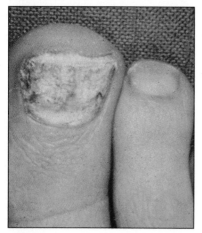

446

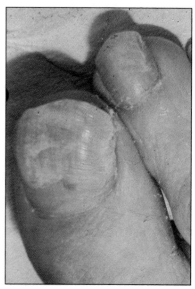

447

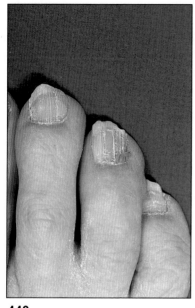

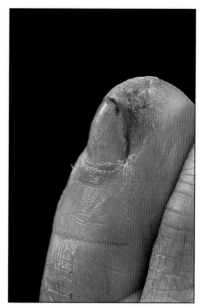

448　　　　　　　　　**449**

445 Onychorrhexis of great toenails.
446 Onychomycosis with lifting and loss of toenails.
447 General skin disease. Eczema of nails—part of a generalised eczema.
448 A small (3") toenail fibroma.
449 Localised eczematous area on lateral edge of nail. Some hyperkeratosis—cause unknown.

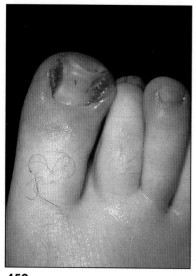

450

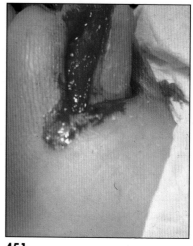

451

450 Infected ingrowing toenail on both sides of right great toenail. Patient's self-treatment has worsened the condition, resulting in secondary infection.
451 Surgical removal of lateral section of an ingrown nail and its bed.
452 Post-operative appearance of a more extensive nail removal of an "ingrowing toenail", as in **451**.
453 A unicorn!

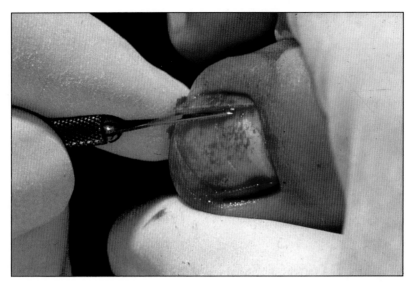

452

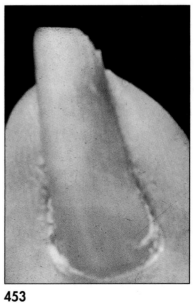

453

Psoriasis in Toenails

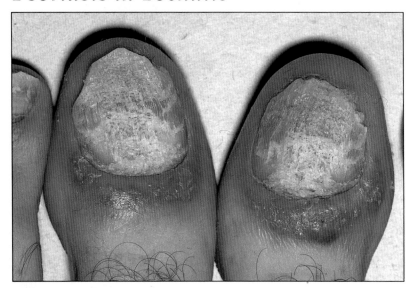

454

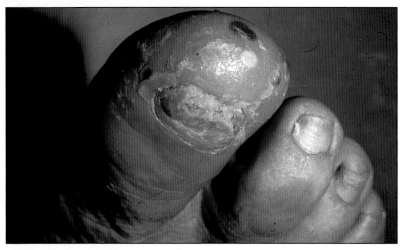

455

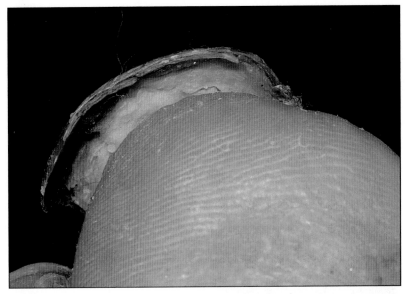

456

454 Long-standing psoriatic toenail involvement.
455 Pustular psoriasis (acrodermatitis), also on elbows and knees.
456 Thickened and dystrophic hyponychium in psoriasis.
457 Nail suggests onychomycosis, but no growth and intermittent psoriasis seen elsewhere in winter.

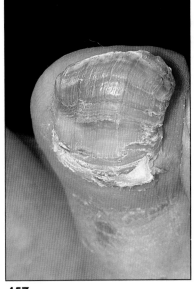

457

Onychogryphoses

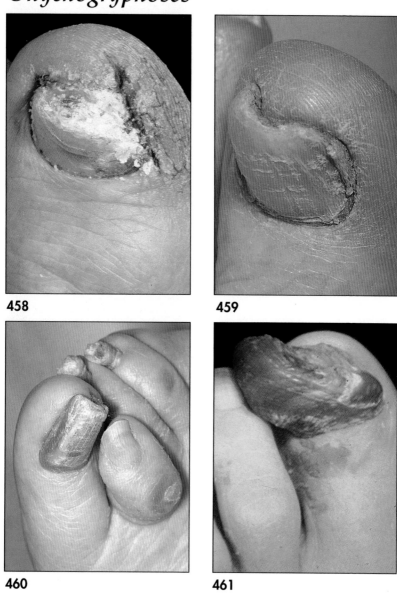

458

459

460

461

458 Treated onychogryphosis of great toe. Note injury to soft tissue.

459 Premature thickening and early gryphosis in a 60-year-old woman. No known cause—due to ballet?

460 Depressed 70-year-old with hypothyroidism, anaemia and onychogryphosis hallux. Note normal second toe.

461 Onychogryphosis of great toe.

462 Treatment of onychogryphosis. Severe onychogryphosis of great toe-nail in elderly man with ischaemia of the foot—also diabetes and some secondary paronychia. First phase of treatment involves reduction of nail and clearing up infection.

463 Onychogryphosis. Note the greenish-yellow colour in the abnormal nail. Skin also shows signs of ischaemia.

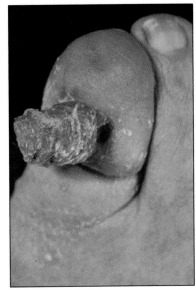

462

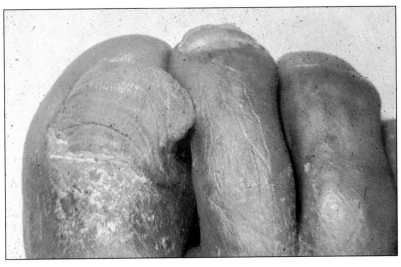

463

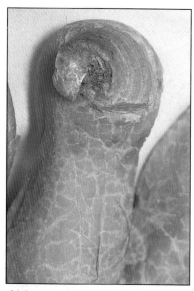

464

464 Ramshorn Hallux nail—neglect in an 80-year-old.

465 Curved toenails of a 73-year-old blind lady, otherwise well.

466 Toenails of an elderly man with no known relatives.

467 Extensive onychogryphosis. Very severe onychogryphosis in a demented old lady living on her own in an isolated dwelling.

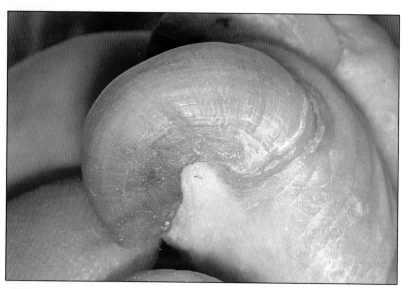

465

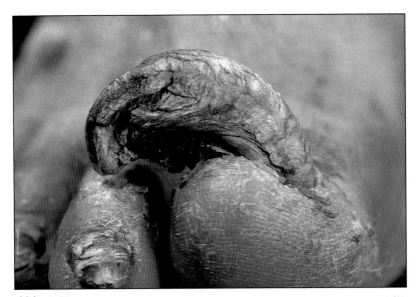

466

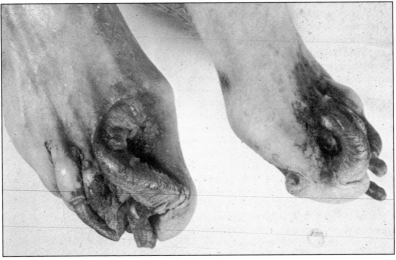

467

References

1. Abramson, C. Athlete's foot and onychomycosis is caused by Hendersonula toroloidea. *Cutis,* 1990, **46** (2), 128–32.
2. Anonymous. Great toe–nail dystrophy. *British Journal of Dermatology,* 1989, **120** (1), 139–40.
3. Baran, R. & Badillet, G. Primary onycholysis of the big toenails, a review of (113 cases). *British Journal of Dermatology,* 1982, **106** (5), 529.
4. Donohue, L. H., Marchese, C. G. & Soave, R. L. Tumours of the nail and nail bed. *Clin. Podiatr. Med. Surg.,* 1989, **6** (2), 373–87.
5. Dvorak, J. & Weigl, E. Aetiology of onychomycosis and tinea unguim. *Acta Univ. Palacki Olomuc. Fac. Med.,* 1989, **122**, 39–44.
6. Jules, K. T. & Bonar, P. L. Nail infections. *Clin. Podiatr. Med. Surg.,* 1989, **6** (2), 403–16.
7. Kosinski, M. A. & Stewart, D. Nail changes associated with systemic disease and vascular insufficiency. *Clin. Podiatr. Med. Surg.,* 1989, **6** (2), 295–318.
8. Mantoura, A., Bryant, H. Nail disorders due to trauma and other acquired conditions of the nail. *Clin. Podiatr. Med. Surg.,* 1989, **6** (2), 347–354.
9. Nzuzi, S. M. Common nail disorders. *Clin. Podiatr. Med. Surg.,* 1989, **6** (2), 273–94.
10. Nzuzi, S. M. Nail entities. *Clin. Podiatr. Med. Surg.,* 1989, **6** (2), 253–71.
11. Positano, R. G., George, D. H. & Miller, A. K. A systemic approach to examining the patient with nail disease. *Clin. Podiatr. Med. Surg.,* 1989, **6** (2), 247–51.
12. Positano, R. G., DeLauro, T. M., & Berkowitz, B. J. Nail changes secondary to environmental influences. *Clin. Podiatr. Med. Surg.,* 1989, **6** (2), 417–29.
13. Rzonca, E. C. & Lupo, P. J. Pedal nail pathology, biochemical implications. *Clin. Podiatr. Med. Surg.,* 1989, **6** (2), 327–37.
14. Sarnow, M. R., Plotkin, E. L., Spinosa, F. A. & Cohen, R. Nail changes in the seropositive and seronegative arthritides. *Clin. Podiatr. Med. Surg.,* 1989, **6** (2), 389–402.
15. Spinosa, F. A., Murphy, E. S., Murphy, C. & Berowitz, B. Nail changes associated with scleroderma, a case report. *Clin. Podiatr. Med. Surg.,* 1989, **6** (2), 319–25.
16. Stiller, M. J., Rosenthal, S., Summerbell, R. C., Pollack, J. & Chan, A. Onychomycosis of the toenails caused by Chaetomium globosum. *Journal of the American Academy of Dermatology,* 1992, **26** (**5**, Pt 1), 775–6.
17. Summerbell, R. C., Kane, J. & Krajden, S. Onychomycosis, tinea pedis and tinea manuum caused by non-dermatophytic filamentous fungi. *Mycoses,* 1989, **32** (12), 609–19.
18. Telfer, N. R., Barth, J. H. & Dawber, R. P. Recurrent blistering distal dactylitis of the great toe associated with an ingrowing toenail. *Clin. Exp. Dermatol.,* 1989, **14** (5), 380–1.
19. Valletta, M. J., Schwartz, E. L. & Tozzoli, D. Nail changes in glandular disease. *Clin. Podiatr. Med. Surg.,* 1989, **6** (2), 365–71.

Chapter 16
Glossary of Terminology

Anychia = Partial or total loss of nails, usually congenital.

Brachonychia = Short nails, congenital (as in racquet thumb) or acquired (through severe biting or hyperparathyroidism).

Chromonychia = Literally, "coloured nails".

Claw Nails = A curving of the finger nails or toenails, seen in chronic smokers (hands), or in poor footwear (small toes).

Hang Nails = Ragged cuticle at the edge of the nail.

Haplonychia = A "soft" nail or nails.

Hyponychium = Under the nail.

Koilonychia = Flattening and eventually spooning of nails (from the Greek word *koilos,* "a spoon").

Leukonychia = White nails—varying degrees or shades. Terry's, Morey, Burke-type or Muechreke's white bands. Half and half nails can be referred to as Lindsay or Terry nails.

Macronychia = Treated onychogryphosis of great toe.

Melanonychia = Pigmented brown or black; can be streaks, spots or most of nail.

Micronychia = Foetal teratogens. Hydantoin treatment in pregnancy and congenital syndromes (C.O.I.F. Syndrome).

Nychos = A nail.

Onychatrophy = Seen with skin disorders such as lichen planus graft versus host disease, etc., used to indicate a partial regression of nail.

Onychodysplasias = Congenital deformities.

Onychogryphosis = Hypertrophy and grossly thickened nails, with "horn-like toenails"—like a griffin's claws.

Onycholysis = Lifting of nail bed either at distal or free edge or on lateral side.

Onychomadesis = Total divisions across nail plate; distal half may then be shed.

Onychomycoses = Mycotic or fungal infections of nails.

Onychoptosis = A "dropping of end of nail" as in onychomadesis.

Onychorrhexis = Narrow longitudinal parallel furrows between ridges.

Onychoschizia = Splitting of the nail plate, either longitudinally or proximally—usually drug-induced. May start as flaking off from nail plate.

Pachyonychia = Excessive thickening of the nails.

Pachyonychia congenita = A congenital defect of the nails, characterised by much thickening, and sometimes associated with defects in other structures of ectodermal origin.

Paronychia = Infection of any sort at side or in the proximal nail fold.

Pseudoleukonychia = Not true white nails.

Striatonychia = Striated nails.

Trachonychia = Literally, rough nails.

Index

NB: Page numbers in *italics* refer to illustrations and tables.